Encyclopedia of Autism Spectrum Disorders

Volume III

Encyclopedia of Autism Spectrum Disorders Volume III

Edited by **Paul Spencer**

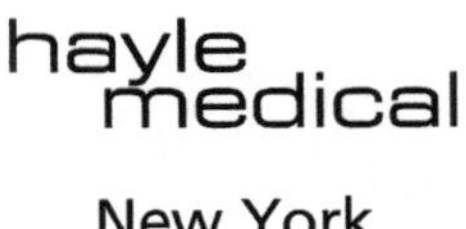

New York

Published by Hayle Medical,
30 West, 37th Street, Suite 612,
New York, NY 10018, USA
www.haylemedical.com

Encyclopedia of Autism Spectrum Disorders
Volume III
Edited by Paul Spencer

International Standard Book Number: 978-1-63241-124-2 (Hardback)

Printed in the United States of America.

Contents

Preface

This book provides a substantial discussion on Autism Spectrum Disorders (ASD) and its related aspects. Many researches are being conducted in the field of ASD and substantial efforts are being made to study it. It is usually difficult for any professional to keep pace with the current developments in this field. This book includes contributions of expert clinicians and renowned researchers from all over the world. It aims towards providing latest information and advances in the area of ASD. It gives broad overview of the topics which may be unfamiliar to researchers and clinicians. The topics have been organized under two sections namely, etiological factors - intervention in person with autism and autistic self & creativity.

The information contained in this book is the result of intensive hard work done by researchers in this field. All due efforts have been made to make this book serve as a complete guiding source for students and researchers. The topics in this book have been comprehensively explained to help readers understand the growing trends in the field.

I would like to thank the entire group of writers who made sincere efforts in this book and my family who supported me in my efforts of working on this book. I take this opportunity to thank all those who have been a guiding force throughout my life.

Editor

Section 1

Aetiological Factors - Intervention in Person with Autism

Chapter 1

Feeding Issues Associated with the Autism Spectrum Disorders

Geneviève Nadon, Debbie Feldman and Erika Gisel

Additional information is available at the end of the chapter

1. Introduction

Feeding issues are prevalent in young children. Feeding will be defined here as the process of ingesting food and drink in social environments where such activities take place. Estimates of problems may range from 13 to 50% in typically developing children, but may be as high as 80% in children with developmental disabilities [1-7]. In 1 to 10% of these children problems may become chronic and may affect their health and development [1, 8]. Anatomical, metabolic, gastrointestinal, motor or sensory problems may be the cause of or may contribute to some of these feeding problems [8]. A global medical assessment is necessary when feeding problems persist, because some medical symptoms may not be recognized as associated with feeding at first sight, such as asthma. Even if the association remains unclear, a high prevalence of asthmatic children, particularly with nocturnal asthma, have gastro-esophageal reflux (GER) [9]. Both feeding and eating, the processing of food and drink in the mouth and swallowing, are also known as activities of daily living (ADL) and studies examining the specific problems of children with Autism Spectrum Disorders (ASD), found that 46 to 89% have feeding problems [10-18].

While these studies are important to determine the nature and extent of such problems, results have to be interpreted with caution. First, small and heterogeneous sample sizes do not permit generalization to the entire population of children with ASD. There is also no consensus regarding the terminology and definitions used to describe these problems, i.e. feeding problem, eating problem, food refusal, selective/picky eating, mealtime problems, etc... Furthermore, authors use different instruments to measure these problems. Caregiver questionnaires are the most commonly used tools for this purpose; however, their psychometric properties are not well established. Further, observational studies of these subjects' eating skills or self-reports from them are lacking. This makes it difficult to compare studies or to replicate their results.

Despite these methodological limitations, it is clear that feeding problems constitute a frequent and significant preoccupation for many parents of children with ASD [18]. In support of such concerns, some studies found that children with ASD are more susceptible to feeding problems than children with other developmental disabilities [19-23]. There is as yet no defined etiology for feeding problems in children with ASD neither is there for the pediatric population in general. Significant associations have been found between oral-motor, gastrointestinal and sensory problems in children with ASD [19, 24-26]. According to Skinner [27], individuals' responses to environmental stimuli shape their behaviors and this interaction constitutes the foundation for learning. When feeding is described as a struggle in the family environment, behavioral approaches such as escape extinction and positive reinforcement are used by professionals and gradually assumed by the caregiver. However, feeding problems may also arise from a limited ability to communicate or from poor social and cognitive skills. Eating skills and mealtime manners are learned by observation and imitation, yet these associations have not been correlated with ASD. More recent studies have found similarities between anorexia nervosa (AN) and ASD, on the basis of global processing deficits, inflexible style of thinking, communication difficulties and impairment of interpersonal functioning and social interactions [28-30]. Hence, treatment approaches used for AN might also be suitable for ASD.

Considering the impact feeding problems can have on children's health, the stress experienced by parents, as well as the impact on social participation of child and family, it will be crucial to continue documenting feeding problems in this group, to better understand them and thereby, offer better treatment. Similarly, it will be just as important to provide professionals with better guidelines to evaluate feeding problems, as well as to appreciate the consequences they have on family function.

2. Essentials of diagnosis

The severity of pediatric feeding problems can range from mild to severe. Despite this wide range, there are no clear indicators to determine which problems will be transient and those that will persist over the long term and may have an impact on children's health [1]. The DSM-IV-TR, a classification for psychiatric disorders, describes criteria for *feeding disorder of infancy and early childhood*; however, this particular diagnosis is rarely used in research or clinical practice. There are several reasons for this. A majority of the children who are referred for feeding problems, in general, do not meet all of the criteria outlined in the DSM-IV-TR (Table 1) [7, 31]. For example, children do not qualify even if they have severe feeding problems but normal weight (e.g. eating foods of poor nutritional value; eating only purees or being tube fed) [7]. It is also not clear which medical or mental conditions, including ASD, would exclude a child from a diagnosis of *feeding disorder of infancy and early childhood*. Other diagnostic classifications and screening criteria appear promising. These are: *Feeding Behavior Disorder* [32, 33], *Avoidant/Restrictive Food Intake Disorder* [34] and *Feeding Disorder* [35-37], the *Wolfson Diagnostic Criteria* [38] and the framework proposed by Davies et al.[39].

Criterion A. Feeding disturbance as manifested by persistent failure to eat adequately with significant failure to gain weight or significant loss of weight over at least 1 month.
Criterion B. The disturbance is not due to an associated gastrointestinal or other general medical condition (e.g. esophageal reflux).
Criterion C. The disturbance is not better accounted for by another mental disorder (e.g., Rumination Disorder) or by lack of available food.
Criterion D. The onset is before age 6 years.

Table 1. Diagnostic Criteria for *Feeding Disorder of Infancy or Early Childhood* from the DSM-IV-TR [31]

2.1. DC: 0-3R and Proposed DSM-V

Feeding Behavior Disorder [32] applies «when the child does not regulate his feeding in accordance with physiological feelings of hunger or fullness» and comprises six categories to be described below. The future DSM-V [34] *Avoidant/Restrictive Food Intake Disorder* will include a description of three main subtypes that will map onto the first three categories of the DC:0-3R [32]. The reader is referred to the APA DSM-V website for further details on the inclusion criteria [34]. A clarification has been made to consider severe feeding problems, when they exceed what is normally expected with a concurrent medical condition or another mental disorder, which may include ASD [34]. The criterion has been further modified to also include children that do not loose or fail to gain weight.

2.1.1. Infantile anorexia

The central problem of infantile anorexia is a lack of appetite, as manifested by a lack of interest in eating and food refusal, and issues of control and autonomy that may exist between the parent and the child [33, 35]. Parent recall indicates that the child will be easily distracted by environmental stimuli, which interfere with nursing from the bottle or breast from the very first weeks of life. Later, children in this category never complain of hunger and are satisfied with only a few bites. Parents worry when their child does not eat enough and often try different strategies to encourage their child to eat. Early on distraction manoeuvres may work, but they do not last, and parents are forced to invent new strategies to entice their child to eat. They may coax the child and sometimes use force-feeding. Despite these efforts the child does not eat enough to maintain normal growth, which may later lead to malnutrition, but will come to attention when the child does not follow his expected growth curve.

2.1.2. Sensory food aversions

In contrast to *infantile anorexia,* children with sensory based feeding problems are not lacking in appetite and eat an adequate diet as long as it meets their preferences which are consistent and stable over time [33]. These food preferences may be based on food texture, taste, smell, temperature or appearance. Sensory aversions may range from mild to severe, with some children refusing only a few items and others a whole food category. The varying intensities of these aversive reactions may lead to food refusals that may get generalized to foods with similar characteristics or to all new foods. Some children are so sensitive to the sensory characteristics of the rejected food that they will not eat any other food that comes in contact with the refused food, or refuse that certain foods be placed in their line of vision, or refuse to eat when others, seated next to them, eat a food that has been rejected or it may trigger an aversive reaction (Figure 1). What distinguishes *Sensory Food Aversions* from normal food preferences is the degree of severity of the food refusal and the presence of nutritional deficiencies or oral-motor delays arising from a lack of exposure to more demanding food textures [33]. Some studies have shown a significant relationship between food selectivity or mealtime problems and problems with sensory modulation [26, 40].

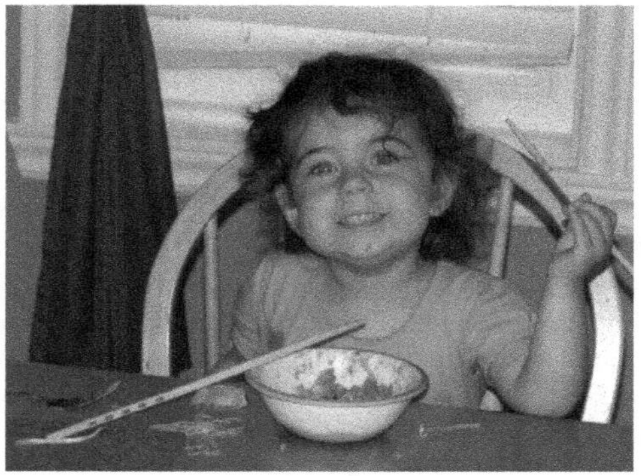

Figure 1. Children learn about food through exploration with their senses

2.1.3. Feeding disorders associated with insults to the gastrointestinal tract

This diagnosis, later renamed *posttraumatic feeding disorders* by Chatoor [33], has a sudden onset and results in severe food refusal. Young children with this diagnosis refuse to be fed, and often cry, hyper-extend their trunk and refuse to open their mouth when food is offered. Posttraumatic feeding problems are the result of a traumatic event or chronic, repeated traumatic events that affect the oropharynx or the esophagus. The event may have been aspiration of solid food into the trachea, related to force-feeding, due to medical procedures, such as placement of a nasogastric tube or enteral feeding. The refusal of food may manifest itself in different ways, depending on the type of feeding that is associated with the trauma. Depending further on the situation where the trauma occurred, such as the location or the positioning associated with feeding, the child may show signs of anxiety and marked distress at the approach of the bottle or the spoon, or when the food is placed in the mouth. Fear will override any sense of hunger and the effects on the child's health may vary, depending on the duration and extent of the food refusal, and the adequacy and adaptations made for nutritional compensation. If the food refusal extends over a prolonged period of time, delay in oral-motor skills, or overall development may be the result [33].

2.1.4. Feeding disorder associated with concurrent medical conditions

The DC: 0-3R [32] also lists feeding problems that are associated with medical conditions whereas the DSM-V [34] will only deal with mental health issues, not medical problems. Children with medical conditions and associated feeding problems are able to initiate eating; however, they may soon show signs of distress and/or fatigue and may not be able to finish their meal [33]. This inability may vary according to the severity of the medical condition. Heart and respiratory problems, as well as allergies and gastro-esophageal reflux are frequently associated with this type of feeding disability. Resolving the medical issues often improves the feeding related problems, although the latter may not always be eliminated completely. Several symptoms such as gagging, lack of appetite, food refusals, weight loss or growth faltering, may also be found in conjunction with other medical diagnoses. It is essential therefore, that children with feeding problems be carefully examined for associated medical problems.

2.1.5. Feeding disorder of state regulation

This feeding disorder is characterized by its onset in infancy, difficulty in establishing a quiet alert state necessary for feeding, weight loss, and absence of any medical condition that could explain these problems. This disturbance in state regulation, similar to disturbances in sleep or crying, will not be included in the next issue of the DSM-V [34]. Feeding is the first competent motor skill of infants [41] and is also an early indicator of self-regulation [33]. Therefore, specific aspects of feeding problems that also coincide with the behavior characteristics of ASD, might become 'red flags' for its diagnosis. Infants must be alert and able to maintain a calm state during feeding right from birth, i.e. the infant should not fall asleep at the onset of feeding, be too agitated or too distressed to feed [33]. Infants triple their body weight in the first year of life [41]. Therefore, a child who does not gain weight will not be able to maintain his established growth curve, or tends to cross over into a lower growth curve, which is interpreted as 'losing weight'. Mother and infant are 'mutual caregivers' [42]; the child who engages the mother visually, smiles or babbles and gains weight provides feedback to the mother that she is 'doing a good job', whereas a child who is colicky, cries, arches away from the mother and does not seem to eat enough causes the mother to worry and to try to compensate. She may feed the child more frequently than a child who eats well and she will also feed the child longer to compensate for the emerging weight loss [43]. The recent development of the P.O.P.S.I.C.L.E Center Infant and Child Feeding Questionnaire© (Parent Organized Partnerships Supporting Infants and Children Learning to Eat), an age-specific questionnaire available on the web, gives parents information regarding typical feeding development and helps them identify whether referral to a health professional (feeding specialist) is indicated [44]. Future studies will need to determine whether the constellation of early weight loss, lack of reciprocity, and distractibility during feeding may be an early indicator of ASD.

2.1.6. *Feeding disorder of caregiver-infant reciprocity*

Feeding disorders of caregiver-infant reciprocity have their onset in the infant's first year of life and may come to attention through a problem that needs medical attention. The infant's developmental progression shows growth retardation and a lack of age appropriate engagement with the primary caregiver. Careful examination of the child-family relationships often point toward child neglect that may have its origin in the caregiver's history. These difficult problems will need to be addressed in conjunction with the original feeding problems of the infant [33]. In the DSM-V, this problem will be classifiable under a V code (i.e. a relational problem) [34].

2.2. Feeding Disorders as classified by Dovey and collaborators

The classification by Dovey et al. [35, 36] is built on an older classification by Chatoor and Ganiban [45]. Of the five types of feeding disorder, which will be further described below, four are similar to the classifications mentioned above. *Learning-dependant food refusal* is added and will include many children seen briefly in clinical practice. In their decision-making model [36, 37], *Autism-Related Food Refusal* is mentioned as a distinct category, but not further elaborated. In an earlier paper Dovey et al. [35] briefly describe feeding problems associated with ASD and touch upon the importance of the cognitive and social aspects of these problems. However, at that time, the authors seemed to include *Autism-Related Food Refusal* in their *selective food refusal* category. For clarity we will present a brief definition of the *Autism-Related Food Refusal* as a sixth category in this chapter.

2.2.1. *Medical complications-related food refusal*

Similar to the *Feeding Disorder Associated with Concurrent Medical Conditions* [32], food refusal is associated with one or more medical conditions. Medical professionals (e.g. gastroenterologist, general practitioner, health visitor, etc.) are needed to address these issues. The child may lack developmentally appropriate experiences with food because of major medical interventions that may have required nasogastric tube feeding which is often followed by gastrostomy feeding until the medical issues are resolved. Periods of longer than 1 week of tube feeding put the child at risk for 'oral deprivation,' i.e. they deprive the child of the daily practice of oral behaviors which in turn seem to have a detrimental effect on the associated brain development [46, 47]. If it occurs in infancy children will experience great difficulty in making the transition to oral feeding. If children have had oral feeding experience before intubation there will be a transition time where they will have 'to learn to eat' again, but the transition will be shorter than in infants who have not had any feeding experience [46]. Dovey et al. [35] describe these children as not interested in eating but generally as happy to explore and play with food. Food refusal can also be present due to an association of food and/or eating with pain or discomfort. Many children who were tub-fed for extended periods will require additional support when making the transition to oral feeding [48].

2.2.2. *Learning-dependent food refusal*

According to Dovey et al. [35], the feeding disorder defined in this category is «completely dependent on the child's experience with it (eating)». Children in this category may have temper tantrums when new foods are offered to them and the usual response of the parent is to take their plate away and replace it with something they know their child will eat. Eventually, parents adapt the family menu to better fit their child's preferences and avoid unfamiliar foods or ones they know will trigger aversive reactions. Children between 2 and 6 years of age often refuse to taste new foods, which generally improves as the children get older. Food refusal based on novelty is called food neophobia and is considered an evolved behavior from human ancestry that protects the organisms from poisoning, at a time when children begin to leave their parents' supervision and gain more autonomy [35]. Repeated exposure, a positive experience and social influence will help children to overcome food neophobia. Therefore, caregiver education will be the first strategy to use when a learning dependent feeding disorder is suspected and rapid change can be expected.

2.2.3. *Selective food refusal*

Initially the picture of the «selective child» will be similar to learning dependent food refusal but for various reasons will evolve into a significant decrease in dietary variety. Here, exposure and social facilitation will have little to no effect on food acceptance and the child will not play with food. His diet will rely mostly on hedonic foods, e.g. foods that have a high salt, sugar and fat content. The child may eventually develop gastrointestinal problems as a result of a lack of fiber in his diet. Similar to Chatoor's Sensory Food Aversion category [33], these children have some sensory sensitivities, both tactile and/or oral defensiveness. Enlargement of dietary variety is a long process for children in this category and needs collaboration of parents, other caregivers and professionals. Dovey et al. [35] suggest that children in this category be referred for diagnostic work-up because of the high prevalence of sensory problems in the ASD population.

2.2.4. *Appetite-awareness-autonomy-based food refusal*

This category is the same as Infantile Anorexia described earlier by Chatoor and her colleagues [33] and is included in the above classification. The reader is referred to it for further details.

2.2.5. *Fear-based food refusal*

Fear-Based Food Refusal is also called Food Phobia. This category is identical to Posttraumatic Feeding Disorders of Infancy [33]. Some authors believe that, for many of these children, food phobia might be associated with a more general anxiety or affective disorder [49]. Food refusal in this category can be distinguished from other categories by the intensity of the emotional reaction when the child is asked to eat the target food.

2.2.6. *Autism-related food refusal*

Dovey et al. [35] describe children with ASD and feeding problems as having «seemingly illogical rules around what constitutes an acceptable meal». We are not aware of any studies that have examined these children's rationale for their eating behaviors and the cognitive decisions that have led to them. Although, we do not know whether Dovey and collaborators have studied these, they acknowledge that these children must make decisions whether to eat something or not. This constitutes an important gap in our understanding of these children's feeding behavior and has important consequences on how we treat them. We observe children's behaviors and decide to manipulate them without understanding the underlying rationale that has led to these behaviors. An interpretation based on the hyper-systematization theory of Baron-Cohen et al. [50] will be discussed in the intervention section of this chapter. Meanwhile, perhaps one approach would be to study adults with autism and/or higher functioning children with ASD where some communication and insight is present, in order to access this very challenging domain. Even here, we must be sensitive to the fact that many other domains of ADL might be affected, besides eating, and that children and their family must be treated holistically.

2.3. The 'Wolfson group' diagnostic criteria of infantile feeding disorders

The 'Wolfson Group', a collaboration of medical professionals from Israel, has studied infantile feeding problems for a number of years [38, 51, 52] and has shown considerable success in discriminating between infantile feeding disorders (non-organic) and medically based feeding problems (organic). Levine et al. [38] compared the diagnostic criteria of the Wolfson group to DC: 0-3R [32], and the DSM-IV [31] classifications in a group of children referred for food refusal. Results discriminated 100%, 77% and 47% respectively. The Wolfson criteria (Table 2) successfully identified a substantial proportion of treatable patients that the two other existing classifications could not identify [38].

1. Persistent food refusal "/>1 month
2. Absence of obvious organic disease leading to food refusal or lack of response to medical treatment of an organic disease
3. Age of onset <2 years, age at presentation <6 years
4. Presence of at least one of the following: a. Pathological feeding or b. Anticipatory gagging

Table 2. The Wolfson Diagnostic Criteria

2.4. Davies and collaborators' framework for classification

Finally, another convincing argument for a reconceptualization of diagnostic criteria of feeding problems has been advanced by Davies and collaborators [39], suggesting that feeding problems are the result of a relational disorder of the child in his social context. The authors propose that feeding problems be diagnosed along 6 axes that define 1) a feeding disorder between parent and child, characterized by the child's persistent failure to eat foods in accordance with his developmental stage and the cultural or sub-cultural expectations. 2) a character/developmental disorder of parent and/or child, where the feeding relationship may be disrupted due to the caregivers' own psychopathology or life demands, and/or where the child may have a difficult temperament or medical and developmental issues that interfere with feeding, 3) This axis describes medical disorders of parent and/or child, that need to be addressed before feeding problems can be resolved 4) psychosocial stressors need to be identified "through use of the multi-axial diagnosis, to reflect the multi-determined nature of feeding disorders" 5) global functioning of parent and child will be examined separately for each, and 6) the global parent-infant relationship is classified through assessment of the quality of the parent-child relationship.

2.5. Parent reported feeding problems

A systematic literature review of feeding problems reported by parents, shows that many symptoms are similar to those associated with sensory feeding problems [4, 5, 10, 11, 14, 17, 20, 26, 53-55]. The peculiar ways in which sensory input is treated by persons with ASD are well documented in the literature [56-59]. The most frequently mentioned problems are texture, color, and smell selectivity, refusal of new foods, and food refusals in general. These problems were not associated with weight loss in a study comparing body mass index between typically developing children and those with ASD [60]. One study even reported a large proportion of children with ASD to be obese [61].

Parents' perception of their child's feeding problem often leads them to seek professional advice. In terms of nutritional deficiency, results vary widely [62-64]. Application of standards of reference with different criteria for severity levels may explain these discrepancies [65]. Furthermore, none of the studies reviewed so far have exclusively studied children with clinically significant feeding problems. Within a normally distributed population one would expect some children with, but the majority to be without nutritional deficiencies. Thus, it is not yet possible to determine whether or not children with ASD and severe feeding problems would also have nutritional deficiencies. Some case studies and larger studies report negative health effects due to selective eating or restrictive diets [66, 67]. Therefore, it is always advisable to refer a child to a qualified nutritional expert when the child presents with selective eating.

Some parents report problems with chewing and abnormal drooling even after the child's developmental age has been taken into account [13, 68]. Nadon et al. [13] compared children with ASD and their typically developing siblings of the same mean age and found that only the children with ASD had problems with eating related drooling, chewing, moving their tongue or swallowing. While parents interpreted these problems as a source of their child's feeding problem, this study showed that these motor behaviors were associated with tactile sensitivity but independent of mental retardation, attention deficit disorder or hyperactivity that is often present in these children [13]. These oral-motor problems are often overlooked, because it is generally a small group when compared to the whole population of children with ASD. However, careful evaluation may be particularly helpful for this group of children, because specific treatments exist, and have been shown to be effective for other neurologically based feeding problems [41].

Anticipatory behavior is an early indicator of social engagement. Kanner [69] noted that infants who later were described as 'autistic' did not reach out to an adult who was engaged in picking them up. Brisson and colleagues [70] made use of this characteristic by studying anticipatory behavior associated with feeding. The authors performed a retrospective review of home movies of infants, 3 to 6 months of age, who were later diagnosed with autism, expecting that they would perform poorly on opening their mouth (the anticipatory behavior) in response to an approaching spoon. Results were compared to an age matched typically developing group. While typically developing children, as a group, achieved 79% correct responses, only 46% of the children with autism did so. There was a clear learning curve in both groups, with younger infants showing fewer mouth opening responses than the older ones, and a larger proportion of typically developing infants opening their mouth to an approaching spoon than did infants with autism. These results are consistent with parent descriptions that infants were easily distracted when feeding, right from birth, and this behavior may indeed become an early diagnostic indicator, in conjunction with other behaviors that characterize the ASDs.

3. Evaluation

Feeding at mealtimes occurs as the result of the interaction between a child's body functions and structures, his health condition and some contextual factors (i.e. environmental factors as well as personal factors). An illustration of these interactions, using the model of the International Classification of Functioning, Disability and Health (ICF) is illustrated in Figure 2. The complexity of these interactions may be the reason why many investigators developed their own assessment tool, because existing ones did not adequately cover the domains to meet the authors' needs [71]. To have a complete picture of a child's problems, it is necessary to combine various methods of evaluation and to collaborate with professionals who have different domains of expertise.

There are a number of methods and feeding assessments, with varying content as well as different psychometric properties (e.g. caregiver questionnaires, interviews, child observations). The following review will be selective and is not intended to be exhaustive. For a more complete review the reader is referred to Nadon et al. [71] and Seiverling, Williams and Sturmey [72]. Other evaluations may be performed using standardized assessments if the child's condition suggests additional problems.

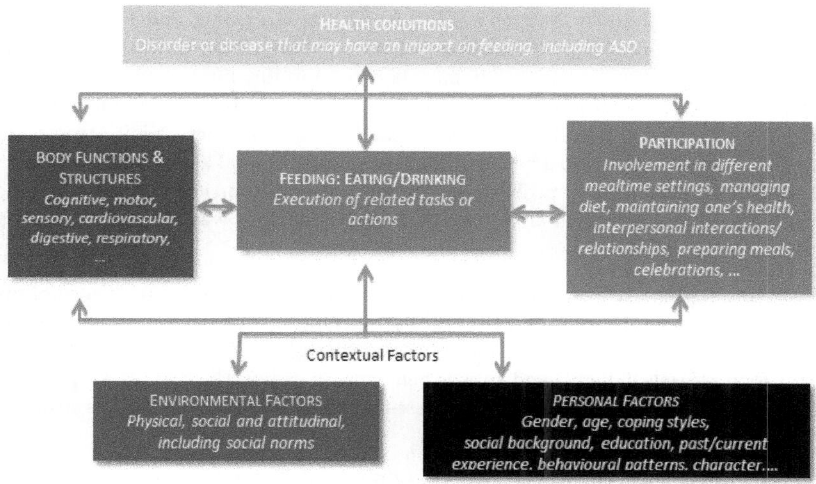

Figure 2. Adapted from the International Classification of Functioning, Disability and Health (ICF)

3.1. Parent questionnaires

Parent questionnaires with interview formats are commonly used [71-74]. These have the advantage that they can cover an extended period of the child's life. As well, documenting the feeding history during the first year of life, and again around 18 months when most of the problems become apparent, sheds light on the evolution of the presenting problems. Parents can provide a more complete picture of the child's feeding behaviors because they usually provide their child's daily meals. The advantage for the evaluator is that he is not dependent on a single meal observation that may not be representative of the daily routine in the home. It is also very important to get to know parents' motivation for consultation, their perception of the problems and their priorities for resolving them. It is important likewise, to learn what strategies parents have tried to solve the feeding problems and how the child reacted to them [75]. A detailed description of the child's food preferences is in order to determine the adequacy of the nutritional content. As well, common sensory characteristics of his preferred and non-preferred foods need to be assessed (color, texture, consistency, taste, smell, appearance,…) to better understand the nature of the problem and assist in the formulation of a treatment plan [76]. A sensory profile of the child is essential and, to understand his way of communicating, his motor abilities, learning strategies, and his cognitive and sensory information processing. It is also important to assess whether the child has a minimal understanding of negotiation, and what his play skills and interests are. These abilities will determine how best to approach his treatment.

3.2. Mealtime behavior questionnaires

The Children's Eating Behavior Inventory (CEBI-R) [77] covers eating and behavioral problems at mealtimes in 2 groups: typically developing children (non-clinic) and a « clinic » group, aged 2 to 12 years. It uses a 5 point Likert scale to identify whether a problem occurs between « never » and « always », and a dichotomized scale for parents to note whether the behavior is perceived as a problem or not. Construct validity was demonstrated by significant differences between the two groups in total eating problems and the number of items perceived as problematic. Internal reliability or item consistency ranged from.58 to.76 using Cronbach's alpha, and test-retest reliability was 84 (parent score) and 87 (total eating problems).

The *Brief Autism Mealtime Behavior Inventory* (BAMBI) [73] measures the frequency of mealtime behavior problems in children with ASD between the ages of 3 and 11 years. The BAMBI contains 18 questions based on a 3 factor structure that identifies limited variety of foods (8 items), food refusals (5 items) and autistic behaviors (5 items). The BAMBI has good internal consistency.88, high inter-rater 0.78 and test-retest reliability 0.87, as well as strong construct and criterion-related validity [73].

The *Behavioral Pediatric Feeding Assessment Scale* (BPFAS) is a 35 item, standardized caregiver report inventory that was developed for children with feeding problems, 9 months to 8 years of age, but who are otherwise typically developing. The tool has a 5-point Likert scale and caregivers indicate how frequently children show a behavior, i.e. « never happens » to « always happens », parents' frequency of feelings or strategies is noted and a total frequency is computed. Higher scores indicate more problems. Internal consistency of the BPFAS is. 88. Test-re-test reliability for the total score is.78 in both normal and clinical samples. The BPFAS was shown to have adequate reliability and validity [78].

The 31-item *Parent Mealtime Action Scale* (PMAS) [75] measures parents' actions regarding their child's mealtime behaviors in nine dimensions: snack limits, positive persuasion, daily fruit and vegetable availability, use of rewards, insistence on eating, snack modeling, special meals, fat reduction and many food choices. Parents also provide three-point ratings (1 = never, 2 = sometimes, 3 = always) how often they use each of these actions in a typical week. The clinician then provides specific recommendations to caregivers regarding actions they can implement to improve their child's feeding. The PMAS was developed with a sample of over 2000 typically developing children [75] but a recent study [79] examined it's applicability with a clinical sample including 49 children with ASD. Mean internal reliability was.62 and convergent validity was demonstrated with expected associations between parent mealtime actions measured by the PMAS and some children's feeding problems. The five PMAS dimensions most associated with children's feeding problems were snack limits, insistence on eating, fat reduction, many food choices, and special meals [79].

The *Feeding Demands Questionnaire* is a parent report questionnaire that measures parents' belief how their child should eat [80]. Mothers of 3 to 7-year old children completed the 8-item Feeding Demands Questionnaire, the Child Feeding Questionnaire, measures of depression and fear of fat. The Feeding Demands Questionnaire revealed 3 factors: anger/

frustration, food amount demandingness, and food type demandingness, for which subscales were computed. The Feeding Demands Questionnaire showed acceptable internal consistency (.70 to.86). The authors concluded that different demand beliefs influence different feeding practices.

About Your Child's Eating (AYCE) [81] was developed to document positive mealtime environment, parent aversion to mealtime and child resistance to eating in a sample of typically developing and a group of chronically ill children, aged 8 to 16 years. The AYCE is scored on a Likert scale from « never » to « nearly every time » describing the frequency of the child's mealtime behaviors, the caregiver's interaction with the child and the caregiver's reaction to the meal. While the constructs evaluated would seem to be similar in a group of younger children, validity for the ASD diagnostic group remains to be determined. The AYCE internal consistency is -.24 for child resistance, positive mealtime environment.55, and parent aversion -.37. There is also evidence for convergent validity with the *Family Environment* measure. Other psychometric properties still need to be developed.

The *Eating Profile* [13] covers eleven domains (145 items): 1) dietary history of the child, 2) child health, 3) family dietary history, 4) mealtime behaviors of the child, 5) food preferences, 6) autonomy with respect to eating, 7) behaviors outside of mealtimes, 8) impact on daily life, 9) strategies used to resolve difficulties encountered at mealtimes, 10) communication abilities of the child and 11) socio-economic factors of the family. The psychometric properties of this questionnaire have been studied to a limited degree [13, 82]. It was used to compare sibling mealtime behavior (ASD vs typically developing) in the same family. It showed that although typically developing children also had some mealtime problems (mean of 5.0), children in the same social and physical environment but with ASD, had significantly more such problems (mean of 13.0) than their siblings. Lack of variety of foods, i.e. less than 20 items, an inadequate number of meals, not eating at the table, or not staying seated during the meal, as well as showing some oral-motor deficits were the most significant differences between the two groups [13]. Even after developmentally related behaviors were excluded the difference between the number of mealtime problems in the two groups persisted. These results suggest that the impact of the diagnosis on mealtime behavior is greater than that of the environment.

3.3. Nutritional assessments

The *Youth/Adolescent Questionnaire* (YAQ) [83] is a self-report inventory for food frequency with 148 items to determine the nutritional intake of 9 to 18 year-olds and the average food serving frequency of six food groups. It provides an estimate of the average serving frequency per day for 6 food groups as well as the average intake over one year. In a validation study a correlation of.54 was achieved between the YAQ and 24-hour food recall interviews [83]. Test-retest reliability ranged from.26 to.58 for nutrients and from.39 to.57 for food groups. A modified version of the YAQ was used with children with ASD to quantify food refusal and food selectivity (i.e. 'High-Frequency Single Food Intake') on a daily basis [64]. Although food frequency questionnaires are known to commonly over-report dietary intake [84], they are useful to analyze children's preferences as it is required when using graduated exposure therapies.

Food records are routinely used by nutritionists to measure energy intake. A systematic review [84] suggests that the 24-hour multiple pass recall conducted over at least a 3-day period that includes weekdays and weekend days, using parents as reporters is the most accurate method for children aged 4 to 11 years and that weighted food records provided the best estimates of Estimated Intake for younger children aged 0.5 to 4 years. Cornish [54] used a three day food record to study a small group of children with ASD, aged 3 to 16 years where 8 had followed a gluten and/or casein free diet for various lengths (1 to 6 months) and 29 consumed a regular diet. Caregivers filled out a 3-day diary of all foods and drinks consumed. Nutrient intakes in 12 children were lower than recommended in *'Lower Reference Nutrient Intake'* for zinc, calcium, iron, vitamin A, B_{12} and riboflavin in the regular diet group and in 4 for zinc and calcium in the diet group although these differences were not statistically significant between the 2 groups. The median daily energy intake was 93% of *Estimated Average Requirements* (EAR) in both groups, and did not differ in the contribution of proteins, fats, or carbohydrates. Fruit and vegetable intake was higher and consumption of starches was lower in the diet group. The author notes that parents who followed the exclusion diet found that it isolated the family socially, food substitutes were difficult to find and costly, meals required longer preparation time, and it was very difficult for the child to make the change to the new diet.

3.4. Direct observations

Observation of the child's mealtime routine in his familiar environment provides insight into the family's daily life and the accommodations made for coping with problems [74]. The family may be so enmeshed in this routine that it does not always realize how it has adapted to the child's problem and to what extent the child's behavior or the environmental setting may contribute to the maintenance of problems. By making several visits to the home and by changing different variables (person, environment, social demands, sensory stimuli, liked vs non-liked foods…) the observer gets a clearer picture of the situation. If possible the evaluator should have a discussion with the child regarding his global understanding of eating and his recognition of any problems. If a home visit is not possible, the parent/caregiver should come to the clinic and bring some of the child's liked and non-liked foods. Familiar plates or utensils can also be brought. Evaluation will then focus on oral-motor skills, reaction to foods, intensity of food aversions, and acceptability of food modifications. A systematic presentation of foods was used by Ahearn et al. [10] for children with ASD. However, a major criticism with this type of evaluation is that it does not measure the severity or the problem experienced in the home, because the context is far from what the child is used to. It is more likely measuring the child's reaction to novelty or the influence of different contexts.

The Multidisciplinary Feeding Profile (MFP) was developed by Kenny and collaborators [85] with a group of 18 children, 6 to 18 years of age, who had neurological disabilities and were 'dependent feeders.' The evaluation is divided into six sections covering: I) Physical/Neurological factors such as posture, tone and reflex activity, 2) Oral-Facial

Structure, consisting of 'an evaluation of the face and mouth at rest to identify variations from normal, using surface anatomy exclusively', 3) Oral-Facial Sensory Inputs: a subjective evaluation of sensory and reflex motor activity produced by stimulation of selected cranial nerves, 4) Oral-Facial Motor Function: a series of voluntary oral facial postures such as puckering the lips or deviating the jaw to the right or left, 5) Ventilation/Phonation: 'a subjective evaluation of breathing and sound production' and 6) Functional Feeding Assessment: an 'evaluation of oral-motor skills during specific feeding tasks' examining spoon feeding, biting, chewing, cup- and straw drinking and swallowing. Overall rater agreement, among 3 raters, was 0.83, and overall rater consistency was 0.90. Other psychometric properties such as validity, item consistency and test-retest reliability still need to be determined. As well, examination of the suitability for the population with ASD will be needed.

The Schedule of Oral-Motor Assessment (SOMA) by Reilly et al. [86] measures the oral-motor and feeding skills of children 8 to 24 months of age. A sample of 127 children constituted the original sample, 90% were typically developing and 10% were children with cerebral palsy. Differently textured foods and liquids are offered to the child in a pre-determined order: liquid, puree, semi-solids, solids, biscuits and dried fruit and scored in 6 sections. Scores are based on the quality of oral-motor, mandible, lip and tongue movements. Inter-rater reliability was 0.75 and internal consistency 0.85 [87]. The predictive validity was > 95% and sensitivity >.85 [88]. The age range of the SOMA makes it particularly attractive for use with young children because of the benefits of early intervention [41]. While a diagnosis of ASD may only be confirmed by two years or later, feeding problems are often recognized by parents from the first year. Treatment of feeding problems is not dependent on the diagnosis of ASD. Therefore, early intervention may prevent aggravation of feeding problems with time when not treated promptly.

4. Treatment

Treatment must take the complete evaluation into account, including the interaction of the person with his familiar environment. Feeding cannot be treated as an isolated problem and the strategies employed should not be limited to mealtimes only. To illustrate: the stress a child experiences during mealtime may decrease his appetite or decrease his tolerance for tactile or olfactory stimuli. Also, if functional analysis reveals environmental contributions to the feeding problems, like inappropriate parental strategies to cope with behavioral issues during mealtime, treatment needs to include these routines as well.

Whether the treatment approach will be interdisciplinary or trans-disciplinary [19, 89] collaboration between different professionals is desirable, given the complex nature of feeding problems and the many factors to be considered [21, 39, 90, 91]. The degree of involvement may vary, depending on the expertise of the individuals involved, the etiology of the problem to be addressed or the relationship the professionals have with the parents [89, 90].

4.1. Parent education

When professionals help parents recognize the source of the feeding problem, the course of its evolution, and what contributes to its maintenance, the parent can become the professional's strongest ally, because parents know their child best. Engagement is better when parent and professional come to an agreement regarding treatment goals and parent involvement is essential in a family-centered approach to treatment [92]. If the child is still young, one would anticipate that the child will become more food selective around the age of two or three years, as seen in typical development, and that this stage will be more challenging for a child with ASD. When parents first learn of the child's diagnosis, it may be wise to show them a number of coping strategies (Table 3), in order to prepare them for the developmental food refusals, or to prevent some problems from getting worse. Particular attention must be paid to prevent intrusive feeding and to assure the child is regularly exposed to variation in the menu and presentation of foods [38, 93]. Parents' actions and their relationship with their child influence the course of mealtimes. Eating is not only about food. At the table members of the family enjoy each other's company, the meal, exchange feelings and family/cultural values. When mealtimes are not pleasurable and some members do not feel respected with regard to their needs and choices, the relationship may become affected. When the strategies chosen by the parent affect the relationship and contribute to the maintenance of a feeding problem, alternatives may be suggested and modeling used, to demonstrate different actions and attitudes in response to the child's behaviors. Regardless which treatment approach is chosen, parents must learn it and the transfer to different social environments must be carefully planned. It is hoped that regular follow-up with the family can be established, so that parent support is ensured and that changes can be made when needed.

- Never force feed children
- Never require that children empty their plate
- Schedule regular meal times, to establish a cycle of hunger and satiety
- Include activities before and after meals, to establish an anticipated routine.
- Use adapted communication and/or visual cues to establish clear expectations
- Limit the amount of liquids (especially juice and milk), because very small amounts can decrease appetite.
- Each child needs a designated seat at the table.
- Avoid commercial containers to facilitate the use of other brands
- Praise 'good' behavior.
- Change constituents of menus regularly.
- Introduce changes that are big enough to be recognized, but small enough that they will be tolerated.
- Adapt portion size to the age of the child and to his average appetite.
- Plan for generalizations

Table 3. Principles of feeding

4.2. Nutritional supplementation

Feeding problems may be long-term problems. This is one reason why nutritional supplements may be useful to ensure that the child's health is not compromised [94]. This will require a nutritionist's evaluation, to determine whether supplementation or modification of the existing diet is indicated. These changes have to be made carefully and follow-up is needed to ensure that they don't suppress the child's appetite or interfere with digestion. Another option is to introduce supplements in small quantities after each meal, or before bedtime. Modification of preferred recipes or the introduction of nutritional supplements to a child who refuses any change to his established mealtime routine may present a major challenge and considerable risk. It is best to try such changes under professional supervision because, if done wrong, children may eliminate another food from their already limited repertoire. To increase the chance of success, it will be best not to change the sensory properties of preferred foods and to present modifications as similar as possible to the taste and texture of preferred foods [76]. Fading and desensitizing techniques are usually best for introducing food supplements [94]. These will be described below.

4.3. Behavioral treatment approaches

Behavioral treatments must be based on a functional analysis in order to determine which behaviors contribute to the maintenance of feeding problems and what function these behaviors serve (avoidance, attention seeking, pleasure seeking, obtaining a reward). Qualified professionals must supervise interventions so that no undesirable behaviors are reinforced [95].

A number of studies have shown the effectiveness of behavioral interventions for increasing acceptance of new foods [15, 16, 96]. However, there are only a few studies demonstrating that acceptance of new foods generalizes to other foods or other environments and that preferences of the child have been taken into account [97, 98]. Different types of behavioral interventions are often used in varying combinations [8, 97]. Positive reinforcement, for example, consists of rewarding the child when he shows the desired response. Sequential presentation is a form of positive reinforcement. In this type of intervention acceptance of a non-preferred food is immediately followed by a preferred food. In simultaneous presentation the new, non-preferred food is presented together with the preferred food. Although not mentioned in the literature, clinical practice requires great care with this approach. If parents report that their child can detect the slightest change to a familiar recipe, or reacts negatively to different commercial brands when they look exactly alike, the child may be hypersensitive to flavors. When new foods are hidden in what is familiar to the child, they are often detected by the child. The danger of this approach is, that if the child has limited communication abilities, he may not understand what happened to his food and thus, may refuse to ever eat it again for fear that this problem will repeat itself. It is best not to use this method without the knowledge of the child. First, the caregiver will want to decrease the risk that the child would eliminate one of his preferred foods from an already limited repertoire. Second, the child should be aware that a new food is being introduced, if we want to gradually diminish anxiety toward this food and new foods in general.

In *food fading* a similar approach is used. The intensity of the taste or texture is decreased by mixing the new food with something that the child likes. For instance, one can mix a teaspoon of home-made applesauce in a cup of commercial applesauce. If the child tolerates it, one can add a second teaspoonful at the next meal, and so on. If the child reacts mostly to visual changes he may be a good candidate for this particular approach.

Antecedent manipulation aims likewise at modifying the characteristics of a novel food or its presentation (e.g. texture, bite size, utensil, etc.), to make it more acceptable to the child and to fit the oral-motor skills of the child [8].

Escape extinction is used when the functional analysis shows that problem behaviors during a meal result in avoidance of encountering or having to eat a certain food. Physical guidance and non-withdrawal of the spoon are the general methods used for this situation [15]. The spoon is presented to the child and kept near his mouth until the food is accepted. Physical guidance consists of exerting slight pressure on the chin, to elicit opening of the mouth. Bad behavior is ignored. This approach is very difficult to accept for parents because it can be very taxing emotionally for both parent and child. Professional supervision is strongly recommended, to prevent post-traumatic feeding problems or adverse effects on the parent-child relationship. We do not recommend using this approach on a long-term basis but rather for specific identified behavioral problems.

4.4. Treatment based on the theory of sensory integration

Sensory modulation describes a component of the theory of sensory integration [99]. It is defined as the ability of adjusting responses to the degree, nature, or intensity of the sensory environment [100]. Sensory modulation disorders (SMD) describe responses that are inconsistent, inflexible and fail to meet the demands and expectations of the environment or a task [100, 101]. One or more sensory systems may be involved, such as touch, vision, hearing, proprioception, vestibular, smell and taste. According to Miller et al. [101], there are three subtypes of SMD; over-responsivity, under-responsivity, and seeking/craving. Children who are over-responsive react to sensory input more rapidly, and with greater intensity and duration than the majority of their peers [101]. Over-responsivity can lead to avoidance or aggressive behavior, to escape discomfort caused by sensory input. Tactile defensiveness is part of this subtype and is probably the most documented SMD [40, 99, 100, 102-104]. Under-responsivity describes slower, less intense responses to sensory stimuli [101]. Children in this subtype are difficult to engage, they seem lethargic and lack the inner drive to explore their environment or initiate social contact. Sensory seeking/craving is defined as an 'intense, insatiable desire for sensory input' [100]. Available inputs are not enough for children in this subcategory. They need input of greater intensity. They may take risks and engage in socially unacceptable behaviors, and may have unusual olfactory or gustatory preferences.

People, in general, react differently to intrinsic (e.g. hunger, pain) or extrinsic (e.g. texture, taste of food) sensations. Reaction thresholds and sensory preferences are part of each individual's unique characteristics. However, these are not easy to measure objectively. Some investigators do measure them, but their tools are not readily available to the clinician [105].

Through analysis of a person's emotional as well as physiologic and autonomic reactions, professionals make a decision whether these constitute a SMD or not. The impact of this sensory excitatory state on activities of daily living, or on general development, must be significant in order to constitute a problem. The association of SMD with feeding problems has been documented by some investigators [26, 40, 106-108].

Analysis of the sensory components associated with meals is essential. For a child to function optimally at meal times, he has to be in a calm and alert state. The clinician assesses the child's overall level of arousal prior to mealtime and may intervene to ensure an optimal state for eating. Exploration and tactile desensitization activities may be recommended, such as exploration of new foods through touch, smell, and taste [109, 110]. Some investigators have found a correlation between anxiety and over-responsivity; heightened sensitivity to sensory information mediates the impact of anxiety on selective eating [106]. If the child's anxiety level is too high, it is appropriate to start tactile exploration of familiar foods or items outside the eating domain. Manipulating foods with subtle differences in texture, smell, temperature and taste can help the child feel more comfortable in their presence and is often a preliminary step before accepting them to eat. When these exercises are done playfully they are often less stressful for the child and facilitate participation. Finally, all components of a meal, e.g. utensils used or food textures, must be included in the analysis and can be modified to better suit the child's sensory profile. Despite the extensive use of these techniques in the clinical environment, research using appropriate controls is still lacking to corroborate results from anecdotal reports [8].

4.5. Graduated exposure food therapy

Graduated exposure food therapy is similar to systematic desensitization, a type of behavioral therapy used for specific phobias and other anxiety disorders. Treatment consists of systematic and gradual exposure to the fear producing stimulus (food), the learning and application of coping strategies, observation of the development of tolerance and maintenance of the engagement of the child; finally, acceptance without adverse reaction, so that the targeted food eventually becomes an integral part of the child's diet. Another goal of desensitization is to gradually eliminate the fear/anxiety that is associated with eating and to replace it with more positive sentiments such as pleasure. Graduated exposure may commence with two types of hierarchy: 1) introducing foods that share some sensory properties with the child's preferred food (e.g. visual, taste, texture) as suggested by Fraker et al. [76] in Food Chaining© or 2) increasing the food's proximity, e.g. tolerating the presence of the food on the table - on the plate – observing it - touching it – smelling it - tasting it – chewing it and, finally, swallowing it [110, 111]. It may be necessary to use both types of hierarchy when introducing a target food. Change can take a long time and it is important that the child does not refuse foods that he previously accepted which can happen when familiar food is modified without his knowledge.

Objective : Introduction of meat

a. Kraft Dinner © (the child's preferred food)
b. Other pasta, but with the Kraft cheese mixture
c. Pasta with home-made cheese mixture
d. Pasta with pink sauce
e. Pasta with tomato sauce
f. Pasta with meat sauce

Table 4. Example of Desensitization Based on Sensory Properties as in Food Chaining© [76]

In Food Chaining© [76], the child's food preferences are analyzed in detail to establish a point of departure from which professionals can enlarge the child's food repertoire (Table 4). No studies were found to support the effectiveness of this approach for children with ASD [112]. Nevertheless, it is currently in use in North American clinical environments and several documents addressed to parents and professionals mention it [76, 110, 113]. Hierarchical exposure, based on proximity, associated with individualized positive reinforcement showed promising results for some children with ASD [98]. Validation is needed with a more representative sample of the ASD population [98]. Graduated exposure may be used in combination with other approaches, mentioned earlier, to determine which foods may be easier to introduce first, to structure the progression of treatment, and to ensure that treatment does not progress too rapidly. Some use these strategies in combination with other trans-disciplinary interventions in group therapies as a means of exploring foods through games [111, 114]. This may be an interesting approach for children who have good symbolic play and imitation skills. Other authors have used graduated exposure with more cognitive-behavioral methods, such as in a competition table or a diary to describe the child's progress, or with positive reinforcement or strategies to decrease stress [115]. All children in this last study were 7 years old or older. Some had autistic features, but none had a definitive diagnosis of autism. A self/auto-evaluation scale for the child who has fair insight, as well as an observation scale, are suggested by the authors of Food Chaining© to rate reactions when exposed to a new food [76].

4.6. Cognitive approach

Sensory hypersensitivities are very prevalent in ASD [56, 116, 117]. Baron-Cohen et al. [50] suggest that excellent attention to detail observed in ASD results from this sensory hypersensitivity and that it leads to hyper-systemizing, an exceptional capacity to recognize repeating patterns in stimuli; i.e. recognition of the rules that define a system. This theory explains «savantism» as well as non-social features of autism, like narrow interests, or resistance to change. When applied to feeding, some food selectivity or «illogical rules», like wanting food prepared exactly the same way every day, may be the expression of a strong systemizing capacity; i.e. sameness helps the child build concepts. According to Baron-Cohen et al. [50] a concept is a system and helps to define what items to include as members of the system. Therefore, a child's concept of 'French fries' may rely on visual systemizing (i.e. visual properties of the food are used to categorize: homogeneous light brown, thin and long, in a specific container), or alternatively on social/environmental systemizing (i.e. categorizing according to who is present or when it is eaten: 'French fries' are eaten after swimming class, at McDonalds, with dad). Because the child with ASD is also hypersensitive, a minor change in cooking duration, a different tablemat, is immediately detected and the presence of this new feature (often more than one, considering all the variations possible during mealtime) may no longer allow the child to include the 'new' food in his concept of 'French fries'. This interpretation of autism-related feeding problems could explain amelioration of feeding problems as children with ASD get older, as well as 'miraculously resolved' feeding problems observed sometimes in clinic or reported by parents. When the child understands and has a better global conceptualization of food and mealtime situations, his feeding issues may resolve very rapidly. Other approaches such as sensory integration and graduated exposure may be complementary, because the first addresses sensory hypersensitivity, which leads to hyper-systemization, and the second supports how changes can be introduced. According to Baron-Cohen et al. [50], changing one variant at a time is better to support the child in building general concepts. Another avenue may be inspired by cognitive remediation therapy used for children and adolescents with anorexia nervosa but it would have to be adapted to ASD, and maybe also focus more on food concepts and feeding situations [118].

Developing a teaching method to learn global concepts of food and eating specific to ASD may be needed. Baron-Cohen et al. [119] found an «autism-friendly» way to teach emotions to children with ASD which may potentially be adapted to the feeding domain. Eating and the socialization associated with it, touches a spectrum of emotions. Children with ASD seem to only recognize 'like vs dislike' and not the broader spectrum of 'tolerate, appreciate, enjoy, love, or crave.' Understanding these may also help them to explore and eat a larger number of foods.

4.7. Adaptation of commonly used tools/approaches to ASD

To achieve acceptable table manners, *Social Stories[tm]* [120] may be used to describe a mealtime situation, a skill or a food concept, that includes expected table manners, and aims at helping the individual with ASD better understand social expectations at mealtimes. A Social Story[tm] may be illustrated such that it explains to the child how meals are set up, why one has to eat, or even to explain what table manners are and what is expected at home or outside the home (i.e. formal and informal rules). This type of intervention was shown to be effective in a young boy with Asperger syndrome, for decreasing unacceptable table manners, such as spilling food and increasing desirable behaviors such as mouth wiping [121]. The TEACCH approach seeks to promote understanding and independence by adapting the environment to better fit the learning style of children with ASD [122]. Visual supports used in TEACCH to enhance predictability and understanding of a task would also be appropriate for eating. For example, one would place only a tiny amount of a new food on the child's plate, if the goal is only to taste the food. To help the child understand the sequence of the meal, one could place a visual sequence next to the plate, to illustrate what he is expected to do, how/when the meal will end and what will happen after the meal (e.g. sit at the table - eat foods on your plate - drink beverage from your glass - wipe your hands - return to play).

Use of alternative and augmentative communication such as the *Picture Exchange Communication System* (PECS) [123] may enhance communication and understanding of social settings between the child and members of the family at mealtimes.

5. Discussion

Much progress has been made in our ability to discriminate between constellations of apparently similar feeding behaviors, and thereby establish differential diagnoses for children with ASD and feeding problems [33-35, 38, 39]. However, each new insight gained seems to beg new questions that call for an answer. The evaluation and treatment for these feeding problems has experienced a similar evolution. We will discuss these in the same order as the chapter has been presented so far, starting with diagnoses, followed by evaluation and treatment.

5.1. Differential diagnoses

One of the basic needs for the classification of a problem is the use of a nomenclature that is understood and used consistently by the professionals who work in the same domain. There is still no universal consensus what defines a 'feeding problem, eating problem, food refusal, selective/picky eating, mealtime problems' etc., in terms of their characteristics, duration, and severity. It may be the source of confusion and disagreement in the interpretation of results from research. Therefore, such a classification would do much to advance the field, by minimizing the need for defining terms by individual investigators in the course of their work. Consensus building of this type is usually called upon by nationally recognized professional organizations which in the case of feeding problems will need to ensure that as broad a spectrum of professionals is represented in the discussions and formulation of such a classification of this complex topic.

Several classification systems are currently in use. These may contribute to some of the inconsistencies of results, but each makes a unique contribution, and so, a comparison may be helpful to conclude the discussion on differential diagnoses. The DC: 0-3R [32], the proposed DSM-V [34] and Dovey et al.' [35] classifications have several advantages over the current DSM-IV-TR classification. These are the addition of the constructs of appetite, self-regulation, and the sensory and post-traumatic feeding problems. Despite these advances, there will always be children who will not exactly fit these new definitions. It must also be noted that the authors of these classifications do not exclude the possibility that a child may present with more than one diagnosis at a time. Nonetheless, there are still gaps. For example, much attention has been paid to nutritional deficiencies and weight loss, whereas normal weight gain or over-weight due to hyper-caloric diets associated with high hedonic value from sugars, fats and salt are not yet covered. These diets are quickly becoming an important societal problem. Certain symptoms and diagnostic criteria sometimes overlap and standardized tools are not yet available, especially for sensory food aversions [124]. The recognition of sensory based feeding problems is new and studies will be needed to validate criteria for sensory based food aversions. It is also not yet clear whether some of these feeding problems are specific to the population with ASD, if they are an associated condition or a learned behavior complicated by their diagnosis.

5.2. Evaluation

In the section on evaluation we noted that the age ranges of evaluations vary from infancy to late adolescence. New assessments may be needed if the age range for a particular domain is not yet available. While a diagnosis of ASD is often not confirmed until a child is 3 to 4 years old, feeding problems are prevalent and often come to attention in infancy [70]. Treatment of a feeding problem does not depend on a diagnosis of ASD. Therefore, it can be dealt with as early as it comes to attention. Such an approach may prevent the serious long-term consequences in terms of weight gain and brain development [46]. Whether early feeding behaviors may become predictors for a diagnosis of ASD will need further study. However, inclusion of feeding evaluation at the time of the diagnostic work-up is highly recommended for the many reasons that have been stated throughout this chapter.

We proposed the *International Classification of Functioning* (ICF; WHO) as the model for evaluation, in order to ensure that the interactions between the child's body functions and structures, his health condition, and some contextual factors (i.e. environmental as well as personal factors) will be included in the global evaluation. As of this writing no standardized evaluation exists that covers all domains of this model. Some evaluations may cover some domains, e.g. activity/participation and environment, or personal factors and activity/participation and so, feeding assessments based on all domains have to be accomplished by using several evaluations that in combination cover these domains. Another problem is that some of these evaluations have been developed for typically developing children or children with other diagnoses, and will need to be validated for children with ASD. As stated in the discussion of differential diagnoses, collaboration by an interdisciplinary team to develop a tool comprising all three domains would move the field forward substantially.

Many of the evaluation tools reviewed above are questionnaires and may have satisfactory psychometric properties [73, 77, 78], while others have only limited psychometric properties [13, 85] and need further development. Questionnaires offer the advantage of describing the child's usual abilities. These behaviors are described by a person who is familiar with the child, usually a parent or teacher, and reflects the observer's perception of the child's performance. Direct observations of the child's performance in his familiar environment are still lacking. This constitutes a significant gap in the treating professional's knowledge, because the treatment plan will be based on results obtained from a questionnaire or from contexts unfamiliar to the child.

Evaluation of children's nutritional state is based on caloric and nutrient sufficiency of the diet. These are commonly evaluated by food frequency questionnaires, and by 1, or 3-day food records [84]. Food intake is very individual, depending on the child's age and activity level, as well as the cultural environment of the family unit. To judge intake adequacy, results are compared to established national standards such as *Estimated Average Requirements, or National Recommended Intake Standards* (NRIS). Evaluation of nutrient adequacy (vitamins and micronutrients) should be part of a nutritional evaluation. A particular challenge is the peculiar eating habits of children with ASD; they may be of normal weight, hence pose no major 'medical problem', but their diet may consist predominantly of sugars, fats and salt. Such diets may also eventually lead to obesity. To assist parents in their daily mealtime struggles a number of evaluations also focus on parent perceptions of their successes and difficulties [80, 81]. We are not aware of any standardized dietary evaluation for children with ASD.

Although some standardized sensory evaluations exist [125-127], they cover sensory reactions in many domains of ADL and so, only a few items deal directly with feeding and eating. Hence, the greatest need in this area is an assessment that will fully cover the sensory domains associated with feeding and eating. Preliminary data are available from a study by Tessier [124], but now need to be subjected to a full psychometric evaluation. Common sensory characteristics should include color, texture, consistency, taste, smell, shape, size of a bite, and appearance which may have an influence on the variety of foods eaten. A study of how language and social skills affect feeding ability and the cognitive aspects that are involved for or against eating a certain food may be appropriate to include, since meals are social events. We are also still lacking self-report studies from individuals with ASD who may help us understand the challenges they associate with eating. An update of evaluation guidelines or even new guidelines for clinicians and researchers may well arise from the research suggested in this section and would immediately benefit the population we are trying to serve.

5.3. Treatment

A combination of treatment strategies, based on a holistic evaluation is, in our opinion, the most promising approach to intervention. Regardless which treatment approaches are chosen, intervention based on the contextual factors suggested by the ICF will facilitate the transfer to different environments, maintenance of the gains over time and hopefully further improvement. Early parent education may be critical to prevent the establishment of feeding problems but will need further study.

We have seen that careful manipulation of foods, the mealtime environment or the nutrient content of the diet may lead to some success in the acceptance of a new food, but one of the challenges remaining is that success with one food or domain does not necessarily generalize to other foods or domains. Such progress will probably only happen once children's cognitive decisions/intuitive reactions for acceptance/rejection of foods will be more clearly understood. We have suggested that one approach may be to study the more highly functioning children with ASD or Asperger's syndrome where some communication skills and insight are present. It may also be helpful to begin work by letting the child determine his food preference to facilitate co-operation.

Typically developing children also go through food jags, i.e. phases where they will only eat a limited variety of foods over an extended period of time. One of the authors (E.G.) recalls a parent telling her that his three-year-old son ate only pasta for three months and once he had his fill he 'returned' to eating the well balanced family diet. What this 'fill' was, the parent could not tell, but it upset the family considerably. Therefore, the definition of what is 'normal' or 'abnormal' at different stages of development has not yet been adequately defined. Despite the extensive use of behavioral and sensory integration techniques in the clinical environment, research using appropriate controls is still lacking to corroborate results from anecdotal reports [8]. Most of the behavioral approaches are 'patient' centered and so, may not take the whole family unit into account. This point has been particularly emphasized by Davies et al. [39]. With an activity that is so 'family/culture' centered as mealtimes are, a further challenge will be to integrate the family into our treatment approaches.

6. Conclusion

This literature review has illustrated how common feeding problems are in children with ASD. However, it is not yet definitively established whether these problems are different from the general pediatric population. There is no consensus yet on the terminology to be used to describe these problems, on evaluation methods, and use of different diagnostic classification systems. This makes comparisons of different studies very difficult at present. Some feeding problems are similar to the sensory problems described in the DC: 0-3R. This would justify the use of the sensory integration approach, as well as hierarchic desensitization in the treatment of children with ASD and feeding problems. Updating guidelines for diagnoses and clinical practice will contribute to knowledge translation from research to general practice. Preventive approaches, and teaching parents how to handle feeding problems also seems promising. Further research is needed to support these beginnings.

Author details

Geneviève Nadon[1], Debbie Feldman[1] and Erika Gisel[1,2]

*Address all correspondence to: erika.gisel@mcgill.ca

1 Université de Montréal and Center for Interdisciplinary Rehabilitation Research, Montreal, Quebec, Canada

2 Faculty of Medicine, School of Physical & Occupational Therapy, McGill University, Canada

References

[1] Aldridge VK, Dovey TM, Martin CI, Meyer C. Identifying clinically relevant feeding problems and disorders. Journal of Child Health Care 2010;14 261-270.

[2] Bryant-Waugh R, Markham L, Kreipe RE, Walsh BT. Feeding and eating disorders in childhood. International Journal of Eating Disorders 2010;43 98-111.

[3] Carruth BR, Ziegler PJ, Gordon A, Barr SI. Prevalence of picky eaters among infants and toddlers and their caregivers' decisions about offering a new food. Journal of the American Dietetic Association 2004;104 s57-64.

[4] Field D, Garland M, Williams K. Correlates of specific childhood feeding problems. Journal of Paediatrics and Child Health 2003;39 299-304.

[5] Manikam R, Perman JA. Pediatric Feeding Disorders. Journal of Clinical Gastroenterology 2000;30 34-46.

[6] Mascola AJ, Bryson SW, Agras WS. Picky Eating during Childhood: A longitudinal study to age 11 years. Eating Behavior 2010;11 253-257.

[7] Williams KE, Riegel K, Kerwin ML. Feeding Disorder of Infancy or Early Childhood: How often is it seen in feeding programs? Children's Health Care 2009;38 123-136.

[8] Sharp WG, Jaquess DL, Morton JF, Herzinger CV. Pediatric feeding disorders: a quantitative synthesis of treatment outcomes. Clinical Child and Family Psychology Review 2010;13 348-365.

[9] Molle LD, Goldani HAS, Fagondes SC, Vieira VG, Barros SGS, Silva PS, et al. Nocturnal reflux in children and adolescents with persistent asthma and gastroesophageal reflux. Journal of Asthma 2009;46 347-350.

[10] Ahearn WH, Castine T, Nault K, Green G. An assessment of food acceptance in children with autism or pervasive developmental disorder-not otherwise specified. Journal of Autism and Developmental Disorders 2001;31 505-511.

[11] Martins Y, Young RL, Robson DC. Feeding and eating behaviors in children with autism and typically developing children. Journal of Autism and Developmental Disorders 2008;38 1878-1887.

[12] Ledford JR, Gast DL. Feeding problems in children with Autism Spectrum Disorders: A review. Focus on Autism and Other Developmental Disabilities 2006;21 153-166.

[13] Nadon G, Ehrmann Feldman D, Dunn W, Gisel E. Mealtime problems in children with autism spectrum disorder and their typically developing siblings: A comparison study. Autism 2011;15 98-113.

[14] Schreck KA, Williams K, Smith AF. A comparison of eating behaviors between children with and without autism. Journal of Autism and Developmental Disorders 2004;34 433-438.

[15] Volkert VM, Vaz PCM, Piazza CC. Recent studies on feeding problems in children with Autism. Journal of Applied Behavior Analysis 2010;43 155-159.

[16] Williams KE, Seiverling L. Eating problems in children with Autism Spectrum Disorders. Topics in Clinical Nutrition 2010;25 27-37.

[17] Williams PG, Dalrymple N, Neal J. Eating habits of children with autism. Pediatric Nursing 2000;26 259-264.

[18] Rogers LG, Magill-Evans J, Rempel GR. Mothers' challenges in feeding their children with Autism Spectrum Disorder—Managing more than just picky eating. Journal of Developmental and Physical Disabilities 2011;24 19-33.

[19] Cermak SA, Curtin C, Bandini LG. Food selectivity and sensory sensitivity in children with autism spectrum disorders. Journal of the American Dietetic Association 2010;110 238-246.

[20] Collins MSR, Kyle R, Smith S, Laverty A, Roberts S, Eaton-Evans J. Coping with the usual family diet: Eating behaviour and food choices of children with Down's Syndrome, Autistic Spectrum Disorders or Cri du Chat Syndrome and comparison groups of siblings. Journal of Learning Disabilities 2003;7 137-155.

[21] Provost B, Crowe TK, Osbourn PL, McClain C, Skipper BJ. Mealtime behaviors of preschool children: Comparison of children with Autism Spectrum Disorder and children with typical development. Physical & Occupational Therapy in Pediatrics 2010;30 220-233.

[22] Schmitt L, Heiss CJ, Campbell EE. A Comparison of nutrient intake and eating behaviors of boys with and without Autism. Topics in Clinical Nutrition 2008;23 23-31.

[23] Williams KE, Gibbons BG, Schreck KA. Comparing selective eaters with and without developmental disabilities. Journal of Developmental and Physical Disabilities 2005;17 299-309.

[24] Badalyan V, Schwartz RH. Feeding problems and GI dysfunction in children with Asperger Syndrome or Pervasive Developmental Disorder not Otherwise Specified: Comparison with their siblings. Open Journal of Pediatrics 2011;1 51-63.

[25] Page J, Boucher J. Motor impairments in children with Autistic Disorder. Child Language Teaching and Therapy 1998;14 233-259.

[26] Nadon G, Ehrmann Feldman D, Dunn W, Gisel E. Association of sensory processing and eating problems in children with Autism Spectrum Disorders. Autism Research and Treatment DOI:10.1155/2011/541926, 2011. Article ID541926, 8 pages.

[27] Skinner B. The operational analysis of psychological terms. Behavioral and Brain Sciences 1984;7 547-553.

[28] Coombs E, Brosnan M, Bryant-Waugh R, Skevington SM. An investigation into the relationship between eating disorder psychopathology and autistic symptomatology in a non-clinical sample. British Journal of Clinical Psychology 2011;50 326-338.

[29] Oldershaw A, Treasure J, Hambrook D, Tchanturia K, Schmidt U. Is anorexia nervosa a version of autism spectrum disorders? European Eating Disorders Review 2011;19 462-474.

[30] Pepin G, Stagnitti K. Come play with me: An argument to link Autism Spectrum Disorders and Anorexia Nervosa through early childhood pretend play. Eating Disorders: The Journal of Treatment and Prevention 2012;20 254-259.

[31] American Psychiatric Association. Diagnostic and Statistical Manual of Mental Disorders: DSM-IV-TR. Washington, DC: American Psychiatric Publishing, Inc.; 2000.

[32] ZERO TO THREE. Diagnostic Classification of Mental Health and Developmental Disorders of Infancy and Early Childhood: Revised edition (DC: 0-3R). Washington, DC: Zero To Three; 2005.

[33] Chatoor I. Diagnosis and Treatment of Feeding Disorders in Infants, Toddlers, and Young Children. Washington, DC: Zero To Three; 2009.

[34] American Psychiatric Association. DSM-V Development. Avoidant/Restrictive Food Intake Disorder. http://www.dsm5.org/ProposedRevisions/Pages/proposedrevision.aspx?rid=110: American Psychiatric Association (accessed 24 August 2012).

[35] Dovey TM, Farrow CV, Martin CI, Isherwood E, Halford JCG. When does food refusal require professional intervention? Current Nutrition and Food Science 2009;5 160-171.

[36] Dovey TM, Isherwood E, Aldridge VK, Martin CI. Typology of feeding disorders based on a single assessment system. Infant, Child, and Adolescent Nutrition 2010;2 52-61.

[37] Southall A, Martin C. Decision-making model. Feeding problems in children: A practical guide, Second edition. Oxford, New York: Radcliffe Publishing; 2010. p. 314-315.

[38] Levine A, Bachar L, Tsangen Z, Mizrachi A, Levy A, Dalal I, et al. Screening criteria for diagnosis of Infantile Feeding Disorders as a cause of poor feeding or food refusal. Journal of Pediatric Gastroenterology and Nutrition 2011;52 563-568.

[39] Davies W, Satter E, Berlin KS, Sato AF, Silverman AH, Fischer EA, et al. Reconceptualizing feeding and feeding disorders in interpersonal context: The case for a relational disorder. Journal of Family Psychology 2006;20 409-417.

[40] Smith AM, Roux S, Naidoo NTR, Venter DJL. Food choices of tactile defensive children. Nutrition 2005;2114-2119.

[41] Gisel E. Interventions and outcomes for children with dysphagia. Developmental Disabilities Research Reviews 2008;14 165-173.

[42] Anderson GC. The mother and her newborn: Mutual caregivers. Journal of Obstetric, Gynecologic, & Neonatal Nursing 1977;6 50-57.

[43] Ramsay M, Gisel E, McCusker J, Bellavance F, Platt R. Infant sucking ability, Non-organic failure to thrive, maternal characteristics, and feeding practices: A prospective cohort study. Developmental Medicine and Child Neurology 2002;44 405-414.

[44] P.O.P.S.I.C.L.E.Center®. P.O.P.S.I.C.L.E. Center Infant and Child Feeding Questionnaire©. http://www.popsicle.org: P.O.P.S.I.C.L.E. Center® (accessed 18 August 2012).

[45] Chatoor I, Ganiban J. Food refusal by infants and young children: Diagnosis and treatment. Cognitive and Behavioral Practice 2003;10 138-146.

[46] Senez C, Guys J, Mancini J, Paredes AP, Lena G, Choux M. Weaning children from tube to oral feeding. Child's Nervous System 1996;12 590-594.

[47] Dunitz-Scheer M, Levine A, Roth Y, Kratky E, Beckenbach H, Braegger C, et al. Prevention and treatment of tube dependency in infancy and early childhood. Infant, Child, and Adolescent Nutrition 2009;1 73-82.

[48] Daveluy W, Guimber D, Mention K, Lescut D, Michaud L, Turck D, et al. Home enteral nutrition in children: An 11-year experience with 416 patients. Clinical Nutrition 2005;24 48-54.

[49] McNally RJ. Choking phobia: A review of the literature. Comprehensive Psychiatry 1994;35 83-89.

[50] Baron-Cohen S, Ashwin E, Ashwin C, Tavassoli T, Chakrabarti B. Talent in autism: Hyper-systemizing, hyper-attention to detail and sensory hypersensitivity. Philosophical Transactions of the Royal Society B: Biological Sciences 2009;364 1377-1383.

[51] Levy Y, Levy A, Zangen T, Kornfeld L, Dalal I, Samuel E, et al. Diagnostic clues for identification of nonorganic vs organic causes of food refusal and poor feeding. Journal of Pediatric Gastroenterology and Nutrition 2009;48 355-362.

[52] Zangen T, Ciarla C, Zangen S, Di Lorenzo C, Flores AF, Cocjin J, et al. Gastrointestinal motility and sensory abnormalities may contribute to food refusal in medically fragile toddlers. Journal of Pediatric Gastroenterology and Nutrition 2003;37 287-293.

[53] Cornish E. A balanced approach towards healthy eating in autism. Journal of Human Nutrition and Dietetics 1998;11 501-509.

[54] Cornish E. Gluten and casein free diets in autism: A study of the effects on food choice and nutrition. Journal of Human Nutrition and Dietetics 2002;15 261-269.

[55] Kerwin MLE, Eicher PS, Gelsinger J. Parental report of eating problems and gastrointestinal symptoms in children with Pervasive Developmental Disorders. Children's Health Care 2005;34 217-234.

[56] Baranek GT, David FJ, Poe MD, Stone WL, Watson LR. Sensory Experiences Questionnaire: Discriminating sensory features in young children with autism, developmental delays, and typical development. Journal of Child Psychology and Psychiatry 2006;47 591-601.

[57] Leekam SR, Nieto C, Libby SJ, Wing L, Gould J. Describing the sensory abnormalities of children and adults with Autism. Journal of Autism and Developmental Disorders 2007;37 894-910.

[58] Harrison J, Hare DJ. Brief Report: Assessment of sensory abnormalities in people with Autistic Spectrum Disorders. Journal of Autism and Developmental Disorders 2004;34 727-730.

[59] Jones R, Quigney C, Huws J. First-Hand Accounts of Sensory Perceptual Experiences in Autism: A qualitative analysis. Journal of Intellectual and Developmental Disability 2003;28 112-121.

[60] Emond A, Emmett P, Steer C, Golding J. Feeding symptoms, dietary patterns, and growth in young children with Autism Spectrum Disorders. Pediatrics 2010;126 e337-e342.

[61] Ho HH, Eaves LC, Peabody D. Nutrient intake and obesity in children with Autism. Focus on Autism and Other Developmental Disabilities 1997;12 187-192.

[62] Levy SE, Souders MC, Ittenbach RF, Giarelli E, Mulberg AE, Pinto-Martin JA. Relationship of dietary intake to gastrointestinal symptoms in children with Autistic Spectrum Disorders. Biological Psychiatry 2007;61 492-497.

[63] Geraghty ME, Depasquale GM, Lane AE. Nutritional intake and therapies in Autism - a spectrum of what we know : Part 1. Infant, Child, & Adolescent Nutrition 2010;2 62-69.

[64] Bandini LG, Anderson SE, Curtin C, Cermak S, Evans EW, Scampini R, et al. Food selectivity in children with Autism Spectrum Disorders and typically developing children. Journal of Pediatrics 2010;157 259-264.

[65] Altenburger JL. The quality of nutritional intakes in children with Autism. MS thesis, Ohio State University, OH; 2010.

[66] Hediger ML, England LJ, Molloy CA, Yu KF, Manning-Courtney P, Mills JL. Reduced bone cortical thickness in boys with Autism or Autism Spectrum Disorder. Journal of Autism and Developmental Disorders 2008;38 848-856.

[67] McAbee GN, Prieto DM, Kirby J, Santilli AM, Setty R. Permanent visual loss due to dietary vitamin A deficiency in an autistic adolescent. Journal of Child Neurology 2009;24 1288-1289.

[68] Dailey SA. Oral motor skills in children with food refusal behaviors. PhD thesis, The University of Iowa, IA; 2009.

[69] Kanner L. Autistic disturbances of affective contact. Nervous Child 1943;2 217-250.

[70] Brisson J, Warreyn P, Serres J, Foussier S, Adrien-Louis J. Motor anticipation failure in infants with Autism: A retrospective analysis of feeding situations. Autism 2012;16 420-429.

[71] Nadon G, Ehrmann Feldman D, Gisel E. [Review of assessment methods used to evaluate feeding in children with pervasive developmental disorder] in French. Archives de Pediatrie 2008;15 1332-1348.

[72] Seiverling L, Williams K, Sturmey P. Assessment of feeding problems in children with Autism Spectrum Disorders. Journal of Developmental and Physical Disabilities 2010;22 401-413.

[73] Lukens CT, Linscheid TR. Development and validation of an inventory to assess mealtime behavior problems in children with autism. Journal of Autism and Developmental Disorders 2008;38 342-352.

[74] Evans-Morris S, Dunn Klein M. Mealtime Assessment. In: Evans-Morris S, Dunn Klein M. (eds.) Pre-Feeding Skills. Austin, TX: Pro-Ed. 2000. p. 157-186.

[75] Hendy HM, Williams KE, Riegel K, Paul C. Parent mealtime actions that mediate associations between children's fussy-eating and their weight and diet. Appetite 2010;54 191-195.

[76] Fraker C, Fishbein M, Walbert L, Cox S. Food Chaining: The proven 6-step plan to stop picky eating, solve feeding problems and expand your child's diet. Cambridge, MA: Da Capo Press; 2007.

[77] Archer LA, Rosenbaum PL, Streiner DL. The children's eating behavior inventory: Reliability and validity results. Journal of Pediatric Psychology 1991;16 629-642.

[78] Crist W, Napier-Phillips A. Mealtime behaviors of young children: A comparison of normative and clinical data. Journal of Developmental & Behavioral Pediatrics 2001;22 279.

[79] Williams KE, Hendy HM, Seiverling LJ, Can SH. Validation of the parent mealtime action scale (PMAS) when applied to children referred to a hospital-based feeding clinic. Appetite 2011;56 553-557.

[80] Faith MS, Storey M, Kral TVE, Pietrobelli A. The Feeding Demands Questionnaire: Assessment of parental demand cognitions concerning parent-child feeding relations. Journal of the American Dietetic Association 2008;108 624-630.

[81] Davies W, Ackerman LK, Davies CM, Vannatta K, Noll RB. About Your Child's Eating: Factor structure and psychometric properties of a feeding relationship measure. Eating Behaviors 2007;8 457-463.

[82] Nadon G. Le profil alimentaire des enfants présentant un trouble envahissant du développement: un lien avec l'âge et le diagnostic. MSc Thesis, Université de Montréal, Montreal: 2007.

[83] Rockett HRH, Breitenbach M, Frazier AL, Witschi J, Wolf AM, Field AE, et al. Validation of a youth/adolescent food frequency questionnaire. Preventive Medicine 1997;26 808-816.

[84] Burrows TL, Martin RJ, Collins CE. A systematic review of the validity of dietary assessment methods in children when compared with the method of doubly labeled water. Journal of the American Dietetic Association 2010;110 1501-1510.

[85] Kenny DJ, Koheil RM, Greenberg J, Reid D, Milner M, Moran R, et al. Development of a multidisciplinary feeding profile for children who are dependent feeders. Dysphagia 1989;4 16-28.

[86] Reilly S, Skuke D, Wolke D. SOMA: The schedule of Oral Motor Assessment. London: Whurr Publisher; 2000.

[87] Reilly S, Skuse D, Mathisen B, Wolke D. The objective rating of oral-motor functions during feeding. Dysphagia 1995;10 177-191.

[88] Skuse D, Stevenson J, Reilly S, Mathisen B. Schedule for oral-motor assessment (SOMA): Methods of validation. Dysphagia 1995;10 192-202.

[89] Bruns DA, Thompson SD. Feeding challenges in young children: Toward a best practices model. Infants and Young Children 2010;23 93-102.

[90] Twachtman-Reilly J, Amaral SC, Zebrowski PP. Addressing feeding disorders in children on the autism spectrum in school-based settings: Physiological and behavioral issues. Language, Speech, and Hearing Services in Schools 2008;39 261-272.

[91] Geraghty ME, Bates-Wall J, Ratliff-Schaub K, Lane AE. Nutritional interventions and therapies in Autism - a spectrum of what we know: Part 2. Infant, Child, and Adolescent Nutrition 2010;2 120-133.

[92] Angell A. Selective eaters and tactile sensitivity: A review of classification and treatment methods that address anxiety and support a child's need for a sense of control. Infant, Child, and Adolescent Nutrition 2010;2 299-303.

[93] Schreck KA, Williams K. Food preferences and factors influencing food selectivity for children with Autism Spectrum Disorders. Research in Developmental Disabilities 2006;27 353-363.

[94] Williams KE, Foxx RM. Treating Eating Problems of Children with Autism Spectrum Disorders and Developmental Disabilities. Austin, Texas: Pro-ED Inc.; 2007.

[95] Kodak T, Piazza CC. Assessment and behavioral treatment of feeding and sleeping disorders in children with Autism Spectrum Disorders. Child and Adolescent Psychiatric Clinics of North America 2008;17: 887-905, x-xi.

[96] Matson JL, Fodstad JC. Issues in identifying the etiology of food refusal in young children. Journal of Pediatric Gastroenterology and Nutrition 2009;48 274-275.

[97] Kozlowski AM, Matson JL, Fodstad JC, Moree BN. Feeding therapy in a child with Autistic Disorder: Sequential food presentation. Clinical Case Studies 2011;10 236-246.

[98] Koegel RL, Bharoocha AA, Ribnick CB, Ribnick RC, Bucio MO, Fredeen RM, et al. Using individualized reinforcers and hierarchical exposure to increase food flexibility in children with Autism Spectrum Disorders. Journal of Autism and Developmental Disorders 2011;42 1574-1581.

[99] Ayres AJ. Sensory Integration and the Child. Los Angeles, CA: Western Psychological Services; 1979.

[100] Schaaf R, Schoen S, Smith Roley S, Lane S, Koomar J, May-Benson T. A Frame of reference for sensory integration. In: Kramer P & Hinojosa J. (eds.) Frames of Reference

for Pediatric Occupational Therapy. Baltimore, MD: Wolters Kluwer Lippincott Williams & Wilkins; 2010. p. 99-186.

[101] Miller LJ, Anzalone ME, Lane SJ, Cermak SA, Osten ET. Concept evolution in sensory integration: A proposed nosology for diagnosis. 2007.

[102] Baranek GT, Foster LG, Berkson G. Tactile defensiveness and stereotyped behaviors. The American Journal of Occupational Therapy 1997;51 91-95.

[103] Ghanizadeh A. Sensory processing problems in children with ADHD, a systematic review. Psychiatry Investigation 2011;8 89.

[104] Dovey TM, Staples PA, Gibson EL, Halford JCG. Food neophobia and 'picky/fussy' eating in children: A review. Appetite 2008;50 181-193.

[105] Reynolds S, Lane SJ. Diagnostic validity of sensory over-responsivity: A review of the literature and case reports. Journal of Autism and Developmental Disorders 2008;38 516-529.

[106] Farrow CV, Coulthard H. Relationships between sensory sensitivity, anxiety and selective eating in children. Appetite 2012;58 842-846.

[107] Naish KR, Harris G. Food Intake Is Influenced by Sensory Sensitivity. PloS one 2012;7:e43622.

[108] Coulthard H, Blissett J. Fruit and vegetable consumption in children and their mothers. Moderating effects of child sensory sensitivity. Appetite 2009;52 410-415.

[109] Flanagan MA. Improving Speech and Eating Skills in Children with Autism Spectrum Disorders: An Oral-Motor Program for Home and School. Shawnee Mission, Kansas: Autism Asperger Publishing Company; 2008.

[110] Ernsperger L, Stegen-Hanson T. Just Take a Bite: Easy, Effective Answers to Food Aversions and Eating Challenges! Arlington, VA: Future Horizons Inc; 2004.

[111] Toomey K, Nyhoff A, Lester A. Picky Eaters vs. Problem Feeders: The SOS Approach to Feeding: Conference Proceedings, February 2007, Manchester, NH: Education Resources Inc. 2007.

[112] Cox S, Fraker C, Walbert L, Fishbein M. Food chaining: A systematic approach for the treatment of children with eating aversion. Journal of Pediatric Gastroenterology and Nutrition 2004;39 S51.

[113] Fraker C, Walbert L. Treatment of selective eating and dysphagia using pre-chaining and food chaining© therapy programs. Perspectives on swallowing and swallowing disorders. Dysphagia 2011;20 75-81.

[114] Toomey KA, Ross ES. SOS approach to feeding. Perspectives on swallowing and swallowing disorders. Dysphagia 2011;20 82-87.

[115] Nicholls D, Christie D, Randall L, Lask B. Selective eating: Symptom, disorder or normal variant. Clinical Child Psychology and Psychiatry 2001;6 257-270.

[116] Lane AE, Dennis SJ, Geraghty ME. Brief report: Further evidence of sensory subtypes in Autism. Journal of Autism and Developmental Disorders 2011;41 826-831.

[117] Lane AE, Young RL, Baker AEZ, Angley MT. Sensory processing subtypes in Autism: Association with adaptive behavior. Journal of Autism and Developmental Disorders 2009;40 112-122.

[118] Lindvall C, Owen I, Lask B. Cognitive Remediation Therapy (CRT) for Children and Adolescents with Eating Disorders: Resource Pack. 2011.

[119] Baron-Cohen S, Golan O, Ashwin E. Can emotion recognition be taught to children with Autism Spectrum conditions? Philosophical Transactions of the Royal Society B: Biological Sciences 2009;364 3567-3574.

[120] Gray C. The New Social Story Book: 10th Anniversary Edition. Arlington, VA: Future Horizons Inc.; 2010.

[121] Bledsoe R, Myles BS, Simpson RL. Use of a social story intervention to improve mealtime skills of an adolescent with Asperger syndrome. Autism 2003;7 289-295.

[122] Mesibov GB, Shea V, Schopler E. The TEACCH Approach to Autism Spectrum Disorders. New York: Kluwer Academic/Plenum; 2005.

[123] Bondy A, Frost L. The Picture Exchange Communication System. Behavior Modification 2001;25 725-44.

[124] Tessier MJ. Marqueurs précoces des problèmes sensoriels chez le jeune enfant présentant des problèmes d'alimentation. MSc thesis, Université de Montréal, Montreal; 2011.

[125] Dunn W. The Sensory Profile Manual. San Antonio TX: Psychological Corporation; 1999.

[126] Miller-Kuhaneck H, Henry DA, Glennon TJ, Mu K. Development of the sensory processing measure–School: Initial studies of reliability and validity. The American Journal of Occupational Therapy 2007;61 170-175.

[127] Parham L, Ecker C, Kuhaneck HM, Henry D, Glennon T. Sensory Processing Measure. Los Angeles, CA: Western Psychological Services; 2006.

Chapter 2

Early Intensive Behavioural Intervention in Autism Spectrum Disorders

Olive Healy and Sinéad Lydon

Additional information is available at the end of the chapter

1. Introduction

Autism spectrum disorder (ASD) is a developmental disorder characterised and diagnosed by behavioural symptoms that mark impairments in social and communication behaviour along with a restricted range of activities and interests. ASD is considered a heterogeneous and complex disorder impacting many areas of development including intellectual, communication, social, emotional, and adaptive (Makrygianni & Reed, 2010). This disorder can present considerable challenges to both the individual and their family across their lifespan.

A myriad of intervention approaches have been highlighted to treat this condition. Some include therapies that have been developed by parents independent of any particular discipline (e.g., Son-Rise Program and Hanen). Others are based on biological approaches (e.g., special and restricted diets, secretin) or alternative medicine (e.g., homeopathy, chelation therapy). Some more prevalent treatment approaches are available and differ in their etiological, methodological and philosophical interpretation of ASD. These include for example, Applied Behaviour Analysis (ABA; sometimes referred to as behaviour therapy), Treatment and Education of Autistic and related Communication Handicapped Children (TEACCH), Picture Exchange Communication System (PECS), sensory integration therapy, occupational therapy, music therapy, auditory integration therapy and speech therapy. Despite the considerable number of various treatment approaches to ASD available to parents and professionals, the majority of empirical support relating to many of these programs remains at the "level of description" (Makrygianni & Reed, 2010; Matson & Smith, 2008), and for many of these proposed interventions there is limited or no evidence provided to demonstrate any effective outcomes with their use (Metz, Mulick, & Butter, 2005; Mulloy et al. 2010; Lang et al. 2012).

Despite the many debates that exist amongst researchers and practitioners with regard to efficacy of intervention approaches, one consensual fact that is recognised across the board is that early intervention is the best response to the treatment of ASD. Providing treatment of symptoms immediately will result in more favourable treatment outcomes (Dawson, 2008; Howlin, Magiati & Charmin, 2009; Reichow & Wolery, 2009). Many have argued that this early intervention will allow greater opportunities for a young child to move towards a more typical developmental trajectory because of malleability or plasticity of the developing young brain (see for example Dawson 2008). From a learning theory account, teaching new behaviour or replacement behaviour to a very young child presenting with behavioural deficits or excesses, will result in desirable consequences that impacts behavioural repertoires and learning history from the outset. In this way early intervention for the condition may affect the onset of additional secondary problem behaviours which are often not seen at diagnosis. As such these may be minimised or even prevented (Mundy, Sullivan & Mastergeorge, 2009).

While a consensus that early intervention for ASD exists amongst researchers in this field, many argue that the actual approach applied during this critical period may be pivotal in producing the greatest outcomes and ensuring the best chance of attaining a typical developmental trajectory. Over the past four decades, interventions based on the science of ABA have been thoroughly evaluated and shown to produce effective outcomes in targeting many of the challenges presented within this condition. Moreover, behavioural interventions drawn from this science can produce substantial gains in cognitive, adaptive and social behaviours in this population (Dillenberger, 2011). Indeed, this approach is internationally recognised as the most effective basis for treatment for children with ASD (Larsson, 2005).

Improving the core symptoms of ASD is a common goal for parents and professionals. Reports of large improvements in this condition have been documented. For example Smith (1999) provided a summary of published peer-reviewed studies involving seven independent groups of researchers documenting dramatic gains when early intervention was applied. Importantly however, in all studies reviewed, interventions were underpinned by ABA methodology and theory and were intensive involving a range of 15 to 40 hours per week across studies. This approach to autism treatment, known as Early Intensive Behavioural Intervention (EIBI) has generated much discussion and excitement, and continues to gather momentum impressing on policy makers the urgency of effective and substantiated provision for individuals and families affected by the condition.

Studies on EIBI have reported the following gains: (1) average increases of approximately 20 points in IQ (e.g., Harris, Handleman, Gordon, Kristoff, & Fuentes, 1991; Lovaas, 1987; Sheinkopf & Siegal, 1998) (2) increases in standardised test scores (Anderson, Avery, DiPietro, Edwards, & Christian, 1987; Birnbrauer & Leach, 1993; Hoyson, Jamison, & Strain, 1984; McEachin, Smith, & Lovaas, 1993; Strauss et al. 2012), (3) increased gains in adaptive behaviour (Eldevik et al., 2012; Strauss et al., 2012); (4) improved language scores (Eldevik et al., 2012; Strauss et al. 2012); (5) the need for less supports in school (Fenske, Zalenski, Krantz, & McClannahan, 1985; Lovaas, 1987), (6) reduced autism symptomotology (Eikeseth et al,. 2012) and (7) decreased challenging behaviour (Fava et al., 2012). Dillenberger (2011) refers to the increasing evidence of clinical, social and financial efficiency of intensive behavioural intervention in autism treatment which has resulted in "legally enshrining" such intervention in North America. For example, the Autism Treatment Acceleration Act (2010) requires that health insurers cover the diagnosis and treatment of autism spectrum disorders, including access to ABA therapy.

2. What constitutes EIBI?

EIBI is based on the scientifically applied principles of learning and behaviour, and has the discipline of behaviour analysis (Cooper, Heron, & Heward, 2007) at its core. The approach generally targets preschool children and is provided intensively, often in a 1:1 student/teacher ratio, for 20-50 hours per week. Dawson (2008) and Green (1996) summarise many of the common and conspicuous features of successful EIBI programs. These include the following:

1. the EIBI program should be initiated as early as 2 years and before the age of four;
2. intensive delivery of the program involving a minimum of 25 hours per week for at least two years;
3. application of a comprehensive curriculum or various curricula, focusing on imitation, language, toy play, social interaction, motor, and adaptive behaviour targets;
4. the curricula and their implementation should show sensitivity to typical developmental sequences;
5. generalisation strategies should be incorporated to ensure new skills are practiced and demonstrated in novel environments outside those in which they were taught;
6. use of supportive and empirically validated teaching strategies and data-driven decision protocols (notably those of Applied Behaviour Analysis);
7. implementation of behavioural strategies to reduce or eliminate major interfering behaviours that are an impediment to learning new skills and repertoires (noncompliance, inattention, impulsivity, tantrum, aggression and self-injurious behaviours are examples of some of the most critical of these behaviours).
8. a functional analytic approach to treating problem behaviours;
9. continual parental involvement and tailored parent education;
10. progressive and gradual transition to increasingly naturalistic environments;
11. qualified and highly trained staff delivering the program and
12. the provision of supervision by qualified over-viewers resulting in ongoing review and systematic progression of the program.

According to Dawson (2008): *"When these features are present, results are remarkable for up to 50% of children"* (p.790).

It is important to note that EIBI draws from the bedrock of a science- Applied Behaviour Analysis (ABA). This science constitutes over 300 procedures (Greer, 2002; Steege, Mace, Perry, and Longenecker, 2007) each of which have been tested and demonstrated to produce behaviour change. The careful selection and application of these procedures to treat the behavioural symptoms of autism delivered within the scientific framework of ABA (outlined in Baer, Wolf & Risley, 1968; 1987) is what defines an EIBI approach. It is critical to recognise how ABA and EIBI are interwoven because the science of ABA and the various behaviour change strategies therein, have a very long history of substantiated documentation (see for example Matson, Benavidez, Compton, Paclawskyj, & Baglio, 1996, who reviewed behaviorally based treatments for autism over a 16-year span).

3. History of EIBI

The history of this early intervention approach to autism has been well documented over the last three decades. For example, Matson and Smith (2008) trace the origins of this approach in autism treatment to what they refer to as a "seminal paper" (p.61) published as early as 1973 by Lovaas, Koegel, Simmons, and Long (1973). Matson and Smith argue that this paper demonstrated a visionary conceptual framework for early intervention with ASD.

"The true significance of the study was the authors' efforts to formulate an overarching treatment of children with autism on a multitude of behaviours including self-stimulation/stereotypies, echolalia, appropriate verbal behaviour, social behaviour, appropriate play, intelligence quotient (IQ), and adaptive behaviour" (Matson & Smith, 2008, pp. 61-62).

Trends in EIBI, to this day, are based on this original template involving the delivery of idiosyncratic treatment packages constituting evidence-based behavioural interventions to target core symptoms as well as expansive groups of behaviours. Numerous studies have been published since this seminal paper in 1973 examining EIBI outcomes in autism. One of the most distinguished and considered published papers which resulted in the acclamation of EIBI involved that of Lovaas (1987). This well-reviewed study which reported an average difference of 31 points on IQ test scores between the ASD treatment group and control group, and classified nine of 19 (47%) participants as having achieved recovery (defined as post-intervention IQ in the normal range). To this current day, the findings of this study have caused much debate among researchers with criticisms focusing on particular methodological limitations (see for example, Gresham and MacMillan 1998; Short & Mesibov, 1989). We will return to this study in a later section.

To date, a substantial number of studies have been conducted and published to demonstrate the effectiveness of EIBI in autism treatment. Moreover, six illustrative review papers and one "mega-analysis" (a combination of all of the data into one single analysis) have been published (see below), each providing somewhat varying angles in exploring the outcomes. Steady growing rates of publications on the findings of EIBI in autism have been evidenced and concise descriptions of methodology have appeared to improve in most recent years, particularly with respect to the inclusion of control–no treatment groups and random assignment of participants across experimental conditions.

The current chapter will provide a synopsis of EIBI studies published between 1987-2012. Systematic searches were conducted using the following databases: Scopus, Psychology & Behavioral Sciences Collection, and PsycINFO

The searches were carried out using the terms "early intensive behavioural intervention AND autism", and "intensive behavioural intervention AND autism". The inclusion criteria were largely in line with those of Reichow (2012). Studies were reviewed if they included a treatment group who received EIBI and an alternate-treatment control group who received either no treatment, a different treatment or EIBI provided at different intensity levels. Only studies including children with ASD were reviewed. Each study was required to involve original research that was written in English and published in a peer reviewed journal. In the interest of clarity we grouped published investigations under the following headings: Studies published before 2000 (4 studies), studies published from 2000-2010 (12 studies) and studies published between 2011-2012 (5 studies). We provide a summary of factors associated with each published paper including intake characteristics of participants, outcome measures employed, specific treatment characteristics and group differences following intervention. The following sections provide a synopsis of all studies identified.

4. Studies published before 2000 (4 Studies)

Lovaas (1987) conducted the first evaluation of EIBI for children with Autism. The outcomes of 19 children receiving EIBI, for a minimum of 40 hours per week, were compared to those of two control groups. The first control group, consisting of 19 children, received low intensity (10 hours or less) behavioural intervention and the second control group, consisting of 21 children, received TAU. After two years of treatment, 47% of the EIBI group achieved IQ scores in the normal range and were enabled to integrate fully into mainstream educational settings while only 2% of children in the control group achieved similar outcomes. In this case, almost half of children in the EIBI appeared to recover from their diagnosis of autism.

Birnbauer and Leach (1992) compared the outcomes of nine children receiving EIBI and five children in a control group (no treatment). Children in the EIBI group received an average of 18.7 hours of EIBI per week delivered by trained volunteers in their homes. Children in the EIBI group achieved significantly higher non-verbal IQ scores and language levels. Four of the nine children in the EIBI group achieved IQ scores within the normal range following treatment.

Smith et al. (1997) compared the outcomes of 11 children receiving EIBI to 10 children who received a low intensity behaviour intervention. Children in the high intensity EIBI group received at least 30 hours of clinician-delivered treatment each week while the low intensity group received 10 hours of clinician-delivered behavioural intervention each week. At follow-up, the children in the EIBI group showed greater increases in IQ and expressive language than children in the control group.

Sheinkopf and Siegel (1998) evaluated the outcomes of 11 children receiving EIBI and 11 children receiving Treatment as Usual (TAU). EIBI was delivered by parents, supervised by clinicians, for 27 hours each week. Children in the control group received 11.1 hours of TAU in a school setting each week. Following treatment, the EIBI group achieved significantly higher IQ scores and significantly lower scores on a measure of symptom severity than the control group.

Study	Intake Characteristics								Outcome Measures	Treatment Characteristics			Group Differences
	Group	n	Age	M, F	IQ	VABS	EL	RL		Model	Hr/wk	Treatment Duration	
Lovaas et al. (1987)	Tx	19	34.6	-	62.7	-	-	-	Intellectual Functioning; Academic Placement; Diagnostic Recovery	UCLA	40	24+	47% of the Tx group achieved normal functioning as compared to 2% of the C groups.
	C	19	40.9	-	57.0	-	-	-		UCLA	10	24+	
	C	21	<42	-	60.0	-	-	-		TAU	-	24+	
Birnbauer & Leach (1993)	Tx	9	38.1	5,4	51.3	46.1	-	-	Intellectual Functioning; Adaptive Functioning; Language Functioning; Psychopathology	UCLA	18.7	21.6	
	C	5	33.2	5,0	54.5	51.5	-	-			-	24	
Smith et al. (1997)	Tx	11	36	11,0	28	50.3	-	-	Intellectual Functioning; Speech; Behaviour Problems	UCLA	30+	35	Mean IQ increased by 8 points in the Tx group, but decreased by 3 points in the C group. The Tx group also made significantly more progress with their speech.
	C	10	38	8,10	27	-	-	-		UCLA	10	26	
Sheinkopf & Siegel (1998)	Tx	11	33.8	-	62.8	-	-	-	Intellectual Functioning; DSM Symptomatology	UCLA	27.0	15.7	The Tx group presented with significantly higher IQ following treatment. Symptom severity was also significantly lower in the Tx group.
	C	11	35.3	-	61.7	-	-	-		TAU	11.1	18	

Table 1. Summary of EIBI studies Pre-2000, M, F (male, female), VABS (Vineland Adaptive Behaviour Scale), EL (Expressive Language), RL (Receptive Language)

5. Studies published from 2000-2010 (12 Studies)

Ben-Itzchak et al. (2008) compared the outcomes of 44 children with autism receiving 45 hours of EIBI weekly and 37children with other developmental disabilities receiving TAU. After one year, the children in the EIBI group made significantly greater gains in IQ than the control group. The authors also analysed whether EIBI outcomes were affected by initial cognitive level. Children were categorised as being of normal, borderline, or impaired IQ. They found that baseline cognitive levels did not predict changes in autism symptoms. However, IQ increases due to treatment were correlated with reductions in autism symptoms.

Remington et al. (2007) compared the outcomes of 23 children who received 25.6 hours of EIBI with a control group in which 21 children received an average of 15.3 hours of intervention weekly. After two years of treatment, children in the EIBI group made showed significantly greater increases in mental age, intellectual functioning, language functioning, adaptive functioning and positive social behaviours.

Reed et al. (2007a) compared the impact of high-intensity and low-intensity home-based EIBI. The high-intensity group was composed of 14 children who each received 30.4 hours of intervention per week. There were 13 children in the low-intensity group who each received an average of 12.6 hours of intervention weekly. The high-intensity group made significantly greater gains on measures of intellectual and educational functioning. However, the children in the low-intensity EIBI group did show significant improvements in educational functioning at follow-up.

Reed et al. (2007b) compared the outcomes of children who had received EIBI, "eclectic" intervention, or portage. The 12 children in the EIBI group received an average of 30.4 hours of home-based intervention each week, the 20 children in the "eclectic" group received a mean of 12.7 hours per week, and the 16 children in portage group received 8.5 hours of weekly intervention. At follow-up, the EIBI group outperformed both groups on measures of educational functioning while both the EIBI group and the "eclectic" group scored significantly higher on measures of intellectual functioning than the portage group.

Given the previous considerations, the current study directly compared the impact of existing ABA, special nursery placements, and portage programs on a variety of aspects of the children's abilities. The latter two were selected because special nursery placement is a commonly occurring program offered to children with ASD, which has received little direct assessment in terms of its effectiveness. Portage was chosen as, again, it is increasingly offered to children with ASD (see Reed et al., 2000; Smith, 2000). The portage intervention also allows comparison of a very intensive intervention (ABA) with a less intensive intervention (portage) in a community-based setting. This comparison formed part of the original clinic-based study conducted by Lovaas (1987), and the current comparison allows assessment of the generalization to a community-based sample. However, the intensity of hours of treatment delivery varied greatly between the three interventions and this can make it difficult to "tease out" whether it was the nature of the intervention or simply the duration of treatment that accounted for the differences in outcomes reported.

Magiati et al. (2007) conducted a prospective comparison of 28 children who received 32.4 hours EIBI each week and 16 children who received 25.6 hours of autism-specific nursery provision each week. The EIBI group received parent-delivered intervention with training and supervision provided by clinicians. At follow-up, both groups achieved similar outcomes although the EIBI group scored significantly higher on the VABS Daily Living Skills subscale.

Eldevik et al. (2006) retrospectively compared the outcomes of 13 children receiving EIBI and 15 children receiving "eclectic" intervention. The EIBI group typically received 12.5 hours of intervention each week. Parent training was also provided to increase maintenance and generalisation of skills. The control group received 12 hours of intervention each week. The EIBI group outperformed the control group on measures of IQ, language functioning, and communication at the follow-up. They also presented with less symptoms of pathology than children in the control group.

Eikeseth et al. (2007) compared the outcomes of 13 children who received 28 hours of EIBI weekly with 12 children who received 29.1 hours of "eclectic" intervention each week. At follow-up, the children who had received EIBI showed significantly greater improvements in IQ, adaptive functioning, and presented with less social and behaviour problems.

Cohen et al. (2006) compared the outcomes of 21 children receiving 35-40 hours of EIBI per week to a control group of 21 children receiving "eclectic" interventions. Parents implementing EIBI received training so that they could use behavioural techniques in the home setting. Following the treatment phase, the EIBI group achieved significantly higher scores on measures of IQ, adaptive functioning, and receptive language. 17 children from the EIBI group transitioned to mainstream education settings as compared to 1 child from the control group.

Sallows and Graupner (2005) compared the effects of clinic-directed EIBI and parent-directed EIBI. This study was the only study we found in our search that directly compared the mode of EIBI delivery. All others either employed an alternate treatment comparison or a control-no treatment comparison. The 13 children in the clinic-directed EIBI group received an average of 37.6 hours of intervention weekly while the10 children in the parent-directed EIBI group typically received 31.6 hours of intervention. Both groups received a UCLA-based intervention (often referred to "Lovaas therapy" based on the original study in 1987). The groups made similar gains on outcome measures suggesting that the less costly parent-directed intervention was equally effective. It was found that 48% of participants showed rapid learning, achieved normal scores on outcome measures, and, at follow-up, were succeeding in mainstream classrooms. Pre-treatment imitation, language, daily living skills, and socialization were found to be predictive of outcome.

Howard et al. (2005) compared the effects of EIBI, intensive "eclectic" intervention, and low-intensity "eclectic" intervention. The 29 children assigned to the EIBI group received 25-40 hours of EIBI each week and their parents received training so that teaching could extend to the home setting. The 16 children in the intensive "eclectic" intervention group received 25-30 hours of intervention each week, while the 16 children in the low-intensity "eclectic" group received 15 hours of intervention each week. The EIBI group achieved significantly higher scores on measures of intellectual functioning, visual spatial skills, language functioning and adaptive functioning. The outcomes of the two "eclectic" control groups did not differ.

Study	Intake Characteristics								Outcome Measures	Treatment Characteristics			Group Differences
	Group	n	Age	M, F	IQ	VABS	EL	RL		Model	Hr/wk	Treatment Duration	
Smith et al. (2000)	Tx	15	36.1	12, 3	50.5	63.4	41.9	37.3	Intellectual Functioning; Visual-Spatial Skills; Language Functioning; Adaptive Functioning; Socioemotional Functioning; Academic Achievement; Class Placement; Progress in Treatment; Parent Evaluation	UCLA	24.5	33.4	The Tx group made significantly greater gains in IQ, visual-spatial skills, and language development. The Tx group tended to make greater academic achievements and to be in less restrictive academic placements.
	C	13	35.8	11, 2	50.7	65.2	45.6	38.3		UCLA	15-20	24	
Eikeseth et al (2002).	Tx	13	66.3	8, 5	61.9	55.8	45.1	49.0	Intellectual Functioning; Visual-Spatial Skills; Language Functioning; Adaptive Functioning	UCLA	28.0	12.2	The Tx group achieved significantly higher scores that the C group on all measures, except the VABS socialization subscale and the daily living subscale. Children in the Tx group had significantly fewer disruptive behaviours than the C group at follow-up.
	C	12	65.0	11, 1	65.2	60.0	51.2	50.4		Eclectic	29.1	13.6	
Howard et al. (2005)	Tx	29	30.9	25, 4	58.5	70.5	51.9	52.2	Intellectual Functioning; Visual-Spatial Skills; Language Functioning; Adaptive Functioning	EIBI	25-40	14.2	The outcomes of the two eclectic C groups did not differ. The Tx group performed significantly better on all measures, except motor skills than the C groups.
	C	16	37.4	13, 3	53.7	69.8	43.9	45.4		Eclectic	25-30	13.3	
	C	16	34.6	16, 0	59.9	71.6	48.8	49.0		Eclectic	15	14.8	

Study	Intake Characteristics								Outcome Measures	Treatment Characteristics			Group Differences
	Group	n	Age	M, F	IQ	VABS	EL	RL		Model	Hr/wk	Treatment Duration	
Sallows & Graupner (2005)	Tx	13	35.0	11, 2	50.9	59.5	47.9	38.9	Intellectual Functioning; Language Functioning; Adaptive Functioning; Social Functioning; Academic Functioning	UCLA	37.6	48	Both Tx groups performed similarly on all outcome measures.
Cohen et al. (2006)	Tx	21	30.2	18, 3	61.6	69.8	52.9	51.7	Intellectual Functioning; Visual-Spatial Skills; Language Functioning; Adaptive Functioning; Academic Placement	UCLA	35-40	36	The Tx group made significantly greater gains in IQ, receptive language, and adaptive functioning. 17 children from the Tx group were included in mainsteam education settings as compared to 1 child in the C group.
	C	21	33.2	17, 4	59.4	70.6	52.8	52.7		Eclectic	-	-	
Eldevik et al. (2006)	Tx	13	53.0	10, 3	41.0	52.5	33.8	37.3	Intellectual Functioning; Language Functioning; Adaptive Functioning; Visual Spatial Skills; Pathology; Degree of Intellectual Disability	UCLA	12.5	20.3	The Tx group significantly outperformed the C group on intellectual functioning, language functioning, and the communication subscale of the VABS. The Tx group also showed significantly less pathology at the follow-up
	C	15	49.0	14, 1	47.2	52.5	41.6	33.2		Eclectic	12.0	21.4	

Study	Intake Characteristics								Outcome Measures	Treatment Characteristics			Group Differences
	Group	n	Age	M, F	IQ	VABS	EL	RL		Model	Hr/wk	Treatment Duration	
Eikeseth et al. (2007)	Tx	13	66.3	8, 5	61.9	55.8	45.1	49.0	Intellectual Functioning; Adaptive Functioning; Socioemotional Functioning	UCLA	28.0	31.4	The Tx group showed significantly greater improvements in IQ, adaptive functioning, social behaviour, and aggressive behaviour.
	C	12	65.0	11, 1	65.2	60.0	51.2	50.4		Eclectic	29.1	33.3	
Magiati et al. (2007)	Tx	28	38.0	27, 1	83.0	59.6	2.2 (r)	4.9 (r)	Visual-Spatial Skills; Intellectual Functioning; Adaptive Functioning; Language Functioning; Play Skills; Autism Symptomatology	UCLA	32.4	25.5	Both groups showed comparable improvements. However, the Tx group achieved significantly higher scores on the VABS Daily Living Skills subscales. Large intra-group variation in response to treatment was observed.
	C	16	42.5	12, 4	65.2	55.4	1.7 (r)	2.9 (r)		Eclectic	25.6	26.0	
Reed et al. (2007a)	Tx	14	42.9	14, 0	60.1	59.3	-	-	Autism Symptomatology; Developmental Functioning; Intellectual Functioning; Adaptive Functioning	EIBI	30.4	9-10	The Tx group made significantly greater gains on intellectual functioning and educational functioning, although the C group did show significant improvements on educational functioning.
	C	13	40.8	13, 0	56.6	56.5	-	-		EIBI	12.6	9-10	
Reed et al. (2007b)	Tx	12	40	11, 1	56.8	58.2	-	-	Autism Symptomatology; Developmental	EIBI	30.4	9	Those in the Tx group made significantly
	C	20	43	18, 2	57.8	53.0	-	-		Eclectic	12.7	9	
	C	16	38	-	53.4	58.6	-	-		Portage	8.5	9	

Study	Intake Characteristics								Outcome Measures	Treatment Characteristics			Group Differences
	Group	n	Age	M, F	IQ	VABS	EL	RL		Model	Hr/wk	Treatment Duration	
									Functioning; Intellectual Functioning; Adaptive Functioning; Comorbid Problems				greater gains than the portage group on intellectual functioning and made greater gains than both C groups on educational functioning.
Remington et al. (2007)	Tx	23	35.7	-	61.4	114.8 (r)	-	-	Intellectual Functioning; Language Functioning; Adaptive Functioning; Behaviour; Nonverbal Social Communication; Parental Wellbeing	EIBI	25.6	24	The Tx group showed significantly greater increases in mental age, intellectual functioning, language functioning, adaptive functioning, and positive social behaviours.
	C	21	38.4	-	62.3	113.6 (r)	-	-		TAU	15.3	24	
Ben-Itzchak et al. (2008)	Tx	44	27.3	43, 1	74.8	-	-	-	Intellectual Functioning; Autism Symptomatology (Tx group only)	EIBI	45	12	The Tx group made significantly greater gains in IQ than the C group.
	C	37	24.2	23, 14	71.0	-	-	-		TAU	-	12	

Table 2. Summary of EIBI studies 2000-2010, M, F (male, female), VABS (Vineland Adaptive Behaviour Scale), EL (Expressive Language), RL (Receptive Language), (r) (raw scores)

Eikeseth et al. (2002) compared the outcomes of EIBI and "eclectic" treatment for children with autism after one year of intervention. The 13 children in the EIBI group received an average of 28 hours of intervention each week in a school setting. Parents were trained for a minimum of four hours each week for three months so that they were able to extend their child's treatment to the home setting. Children in the "eclectic" group received an average of 29.1 hours of intervention each week. Following treatment, the EIBI group outperformed the control group on measures of intellectual functioning, visual-spatial skills, and language functioning. They also engaged in fewer disruptive behaviours than the "eclectic" group. However, the "eclectic" group showed significantly greater increases in adaptive functioning than the EIBI group.

Smith et al. (2000) evaluated the outcomes of children with autism or pervasive developmental disorder not otherwise specified who were assigned to an EIBI group or parent-delivered behavioural intervention group. The 15 children in the EIBI group received, on average, 24.5 hours of intervention each week delivered by trained student therapists while parents were included in five hours of teaching each week. The 13 children in the parent-delivered behaviour received 15-20 hours of intervention each week. Their parents received bi-weekly training for 3-9 months and a minimum of one hour of supervision each week. At the end of the treatment phase, the EIBI group performed significantly better than the parent-trained group on measures of intellectual functioning, visual-spatial skills, language, and academic functioning. The groups did not differ on measures of adaptive functioning or challenging behaviours. Children with pervasive developmental disorder not otherwise specified tended to respond better to treatment than children with autism.

6. Studies published between 2011-2012 (5 Studies)

Strauss et al. (2012) compared the outcomes of 24 children receiving 35 hours of EIBI each week and 20 children receiving 12 hours of a mixed "eclectic" intervention each week after six months of treatment. EIBI was delivered by staff and by parents, following initial comprehensive parent training. At follow-up, the EIBI group outperformed the control group on IQ measures, early language measures, and also showed greater reductions in autism severity. Both groups made significant gains in adaptive behaviour and receptive language. However, it was found that the "eclectic" intervention led to significant reductions in parental stress while parental stress in the EIBI group did not change over the course of treatment.

Flanagan et al. (2012) conducted a retrospective comparison of the outcomes of 61 children receiving EIBI for over two years and 61 children, matched on chronological age, who were on a treatment waitlist. Children in the EIBI group received, on average, 25.8 hours of treatment each week, typically at community treatment centres, and parent training was available and encouraged. The EIBI group made significantly greater gains in intellectual functioning and adaptive function, and scored lower on a measure of autism symptomatology. Furthermore, younger age at treatment onset, and higher adaptive skills, were found to predict better EIBI treatment outcomes.

Eldevik et al. (2012) analysed the outcomes of 31 children receiving EIBI in a mainstream pre-school and 12 children receiving TAU in the form of an "eclectic" mix of interventions. The EIBI group typically received 13.6 hours of intervention each week and parents were encouraged to use behavioural procedures at home to promote generalisation and maintenance. The TAU group received a minimum of five hours of treatment each week. After two years, the EIBI group achieved significantly greater scores on measures of intellectual and adaptive functioning.

Study	Intake Characteristics								Outcome Measures	Treatment Characteristics			Group Differences
	Group	n	Age	M, F	IQ	VABS	EL	RL		Model	Hr/wk	Treatment Duration	
Fava et al. (2011)	Tx	12	52.0	10,2	62.1	63.3	33.7	48.6	Autism Symptomatology; Intellectual Functioning; Adaptive Functioning; Language Functioning; Challenging Behaviours; Comorbid Psychopathology; Parental Stress	EIBI	14	6	Tx group showed significant changes in autism severity, intellectual functioning, adaptive behaviour (except for on the VABS socialization subscale), and on ADHD symptomatology. A significant decrease in challenging behaviours was also observed. The C group showed significant changes on all subscales of the VABS. Parents of children in the C group reported significantly less stress.
	C	10	43.7	9,1	69.1	44.3	29.0	84.5		Eclectic	12	6	
Eikeseth et al. 2012	Tx	35	47	29, 6	-	67	-	-	Adaptive Functioning; Autism Symtomatology	UCLA	23	12	Tx group scored significantly higher on all VABS subscales. The Tx group showed significant reductions in autism symptomatology
	C	24	53	20, 4	-	63.6	-	-		Eclectic	-	12	
Eldevik et al. (2012)	Tx	31	42.2	25, 6	51.7	62.5	-	-	Intellectual Functioning; Adaptive Functioning;	EIBI	13.6	25.1	The Tx group made significantly larger gains on intellectual functioning and adaptive behaviour.
	C	12	46.2	8, 4	51.6	58.9	-	-		TAU	5+	24.6	
Flanagan et al. 2012	Tx	79	42.93	69, 10	-	55.38	-	-	Autism Symptomatology; Adaptive	EIBI	25.81	27.84	The Tx group made significantly more gains on all VABS

Study	Intake Characteristics								Outcome Measures	Treatment Characteristics			Group Differences
	Group	n	Age	M, F	IQ	VABS	EL	RL		Model	Hr/wk	Treatment Duration	
	Control	63	42.79	53, 10	-	55.49	-	-	Functioning; Intellectual Functioning	Waitlist Control	-	17.01	subscales. They achieved significantly higher IQ scores and scored significantly lower on a measure of autism symptomatology.
Strauss et al. 2012	Tx	23	55.67	22, 2	58	78.33	32.95	52.60	Autism Symptomatology; Intellectual Functioning; Adaptive Functioning; Language Functioning; Challenging Behaviours; Parental Stress	EIBI	35	6	Tx group showed significantly greater gains in intellectual functioning, expressive language, and social interactions. They showed significantly greater reductions in autism symptomatology and challenging behaviour. Both groups made significant gains in receptive language and adaptive behaviour. Parents in the Tx group were significantly more stressed.
	C	20	41.94	19, 1	66.91	66.92	16.88	47.87		Eclectic	12	6	

Table 3. Summary of EIBI studies between2011-2012, M, F (male, female), VABS (Vineland Adaptive Behaviour Scale), EL (Expressive Language), RL (Receptive Language)

Eikeseth et al. (2012) examined the outcomes of 35 children receiving EIBI and 24 children receiving TAU after one year of treatment. Children in the EIBI group received 23 hours of intervention per week, on average, and parent training was provided. Children in the "eclectic" group were attending special education settings where teachers incorporated a variety of interventions. The children in the EIBI group made significantly greater gains in adaptive functioning. They also demonstrated reduced autism symptomatology.

Fava et al. (2011) compared the outcomes of 12 children receiving EIBI and 10 children receiving "eclectic" intervention after six months of treatment. EIBI was delivered by trained therapists, in a clinic-based setting, and by intensively trained and supervised parents, in a home-based setting, with children receiving 14 hours per week on average. Children in the "eclectic" group typically received approximately 12 hours per week. After six months of intervention, the EIBI group showed significantly greater increases in intellectual functioning, and significantly greater decreases in autism symptomatology and challenging behaviour. Both groups, however, showed significant gains in adaptive functioning. Parents in the "eclectic" group showed significant reductions in stress over the course of treatment while no changes in parental stress were observed for the EIBI group.

7. Challenges to EIBI

Ongoing analysis of the outcomes of EIBI in comparison to other treatment programs is clearly continuing to capture the interest of many researchers with five studies alone demonstrating outcomes between 2011 and 2012. Indeed, given the growing international recognition of EIBI as the recommended approach to autism intervention, this ongoing investigation and demonstration of effects is vital. Such demonstrations and continuous rigor in testing this approach with children with autism diagnoses, substantiates the view that intensive early intervention using the scientific precision of behaviour analysis, can be a very powerful intervention (Howlin, 2010; Granpeesheh, Tarbox & Dixon, 2009).

However, despite publication of the numerous studies outlined above, criticism of methodological stringency and dependent variables analysed within and across them, has been documented.

"Remarkably, despite thousands of ABA-EIBI studies on specific core deficits, and related challenging behaviours and skills, and EIBI studies as well, some researchers still question the efficacy of these methods" (Matson, Tureck, Turygin, Beighley & Rieske, 2012, p.1413).

One of the most pronounced criticisms of EIBI research for some time is that large multi-element randomized clinical trials are required to provide a definitive scientific demonstration of its effectiveness in autism treatment (Spreckley & Boyd, 2009). We, and others, (e.g., Keenan & Dillenberger, 2011; Matson et al. 2012) do not support this view and we encourage the reader to examine an excellent rebuttal of the reasons that the gold standard, randomized controlled trial in research evaluation, is in actual fact inappropriate for the design and evaluation of individualised treatment protocols (see Keenan &Dillenberger, 2011 for a thorough analysis).

One criticism presented in relation to the overall interpretation of the studies outlined in this chapter involves the issue that large idiosyncratic differences occur across children diagnosed with autism. Because of the extensive discrepant features and their expression across the condition, Howlin (2010) stresses the need to determine which components of the intervention work best for specific individuals and under what set of circumstances. Smith et al. (2010) also suggest that ongoing research is necessary in identifying key moderating variables in EIBI outcomes. Specifically, they pose the question of what are the most effective components, and the amount of such components, in producing marked changes in core autism symptoms and additional problems. Other researchers have also emphasised this point (Alessandri, Thorp, Mundy, & Tuchman, 2005; Granpeesheh et al. (2009). For some, determining predictor variables such as personal characteristics affecting outcomes has been a focus. For example, Itzchak and Zachor (2009) demonstrated that the presence of an intellectual disability and significantly delayed adaptive skills in young children with autism was a major risk factor and a predictor of weaker outcomes for EIBI. They also showed that children who were 30 months of age or younger responded significantly better to early intervention. A more recent study by Perry et al. (2011) showed that variables including younger age and higher intellectual functioning at onset of intervention were predictors of greater positive effects. Not surprisingly, Perry et al. (2011) also found that duration of intervention was a predictor of positive outcomes for young children undergoing EIBI- the longer the child participated in the intervention, the better the outcome.

While EIBI programs provide strong adherence to the framework and foundational principles of learning within ABA, some investigators have followed a particular "brand name" approach (Healy, Leader & Reed, 2010). There are a number of different ABA approaches that have been outlined in a variety of sources (some examples include: Greer, Keohane & Healy, 2002; Koegel & Koegel, 2006; Lovaas, 1981; Lovaas & Smith, 1989; Sundberg & Michael, 2001). Often this "branding" can lead to obfuscation for the reader in interpreting what "type" of EIBI/ABA program is best. However, these approaches are all built on the same bedrock sharing important common features- intensity in program delivery (up to 40 hours weekly for at least three years), one-to-one teaching where the individual requires such intensive instruction, and discrete-trial reinforcement-based methods (in both massed trial formats and natural environmental teaching opportunities) incorporated within the scientific stringency of a behaviour analytic framework (Matson et al. 2012).

Magiati and Howlin (2001) have argued that many of the EIBI studies employ different measurements across participants and at baseline and follow up thereby compromising interpretation and reliability. For example, Eikeseth et al. (2002) and Howard et al. (2005) did not use the same tests at baseline and at follow up phases. Inconsistencies in participant characteristics across groups (lack of matching: (e.g., Eldevik, Eikeseth, Jahr, & Smith, 2006; Fenske, Zalenski, Krantz, & McClannahan, 1985) have also been critiqued within the studies. In addition, different investigators examined various settings for EIBI- some were clinic-based (Ben-Itzchak et al., 2007; Eldevik et al., 2006) others were community-based (Cohen et al., 2006; Eikeseth et al. 2002; Eikeseth et al., 2007; Eikeseth et al., 2012; Eldevik et al., 2012; Flanagan et al., 2012; Howard et al. 2005; Magiati et al., 2007), while others were home-based (Reed et al., 2007a; Reed et al., 2007b; Remington et al., 2007; Sheinkopf & Siegel, 1998;Smith et al., 2000). This variation in measures/settings across studies may provide challenges in the generalisation of intervention outcomes to different environments (Mudford et al., 2009).

However, we believe that it is critical to be able to assess the effectiveness of EIBI across participants who may reflect different tracts on the spectrum i.e., those with more severe core autism symptoms, presence of challenging behaviours, less linguistically able; impaired IQ; co-morbid or co-occurring problems etc. In this sense it appears important to utilise a wide range of instruments in the assessment procedure, not only to examine autism severity but also measures of intellectual functioning, adaptive behaviour, challenging behaviour, comorbid psychopathology and educational functioning.

Treatment integrity including initial training of therapists and parents along with continual supervision is often not reported in studies yet many authors have written on the importance of adherence to the scientific rigor of ABA (Symes, Remington, Brown & Hastings, 2006). While many of the studies reviewed referred to training either for therapists or parents, detail on the fidelity of treatment delivery was not measured. Where some have investigated adherence to strict training protocols, highly effective outcomes can be demonstrated using EIBI (see McGarrell, Healy, Leader, O'Connor & Kenny, 2009).

Critiques of the initial results reported by Lovaas (1987) concerning the effectiveness of EIBI were dominant amongst the most vociferous arbiters, especially given that exact replication of such results is not evident to date. Indeed, this is one of the greatest challenges faced by many EIBI researchers. The children undergoing EIBI treatment in the Lovaas study made remarkable gains of up to 30 IQ points and were not noticeably different from neuro typical developing children after 3 years of the intervention. Replications of this original study have certainly attempted to address the methodological criticisms by incorporating more rigorous experimental design including random assignment to groups (Sallows and Graupner 2005; Smith et al. 2000). However, studies to date have yet to achieve the extent of the outcomes reported by Lovaas (1987).

It is clear that over time the methodological criticisms of the earlier studies have been addressed by more recent investigators. Some of the recent published studies have employed larger small sample sizes, comparison groups, random assignment of the children to groups, matched characteristics across groups and standardising measures used for assessment between and within children (e.g., Flanagan et al., 2012)

Certainly, consistency in measures at baseline and follow-up has improved with most of the studies published between 2011-2012 implementing the same measures at entry and output for the majority of variables measured (Eikeseth, et al., 2012, Eldevik, et al, 2012; Fava et al., 2011; Flanagan et al., 2012; Strauss et al., 2012). Furthermore, it is worth noting that most recent studies on EIBI are employing a more extensive battery of measures to assess the effects of EIBI- in addition to IQ and adaptive behaviour which was the focus of earlier research. For example, Fava et al. (2011) and Strauss et al. (2012) measured autism symptomatology, language functioning, challenging behaviour, comorbid psychopathology, and parental stress as outcomes of EIBI. Eikeseth et al. (2012) and Flanagan et al. (2012) also examined autism symptomatology as a dependent variable. This focus on increasing evaluation of treatment outcomes is a welcome development in EIBI research. Examining the impact of EIBI on the core symptoms of autism, challenging behaviours and comorbid psychopathology provides an exciting avenue for future research.

While some authors have provided criticism in response to their interpretation of the EIBI outcome studies summarised within this chapter (e.g., Shea, 2004), others have acknowledged the long-term effects of such an intervention resulting from the best empirically validated interventions (e.g., Granpeesheh, Tarbox & Dixon, 2009).

Prior to 2009 six EIBI descriptive review papers were published each analysing methodologies, variables and outcomes from different perspectives (e.g., Eikeseth 2009; Granpeesheh et al. 2009; Howlin, Magiati & Charman, 2009; Matson and Smith 2008; Reichow & Wolery, 2009; Rogers and Vismara, 2008). As well as these research reviews, Eldevik et al. (2010) gathered individual participant data from 16 group design studies on behavioural intervention for children with autism, resulting in individual participant data for 309 participants in an EIBI group, 39 participants in an alternate treatment comparison group, and 105 in a control group-no treatment group. Their analysis revealed that more children who underwent behavioral intervention achieved significantly greater change in IQ and adaptive behaviour compared with the comparison and control groups (see Eldevik et al. 2010). We encourage the reader to examine these papers in order to discern the conventional acclaim of EIBI as an acknowledged intervention for ASD.

More importantly, since 2009 EIBI research for young children with ASD has been subject to six meta-analytic reviews (Eldevik et al. 2009; Makrygianni and Reed 2010; Reichow and Wolery 2009; Peters-Scheffer, Didden, Korzilius & Sturmey, 2011; Spreckley and Boyd 2009; Virue΄s-Ortega, 2010). A meta-analysis is a particular type of statistical method for integrating results from many individual studies. This type of statistic can be useful for obtaining an overall estimate of whether or not an intervention is effective and, if so, what the size of the benefits are (i.e., the effect size). The overwhelming findings from five of the six meta-analyses conducted between 2009 to 2012 (Eldevik et al. 2009; Makrygianni and Reed 2010; Peters-Scheffer et al., 2011; Reichow & Wolery 2009; Virue΄s-Ortega 2010) concluded that EIBI was an effective intervention strategy for many children with ASD, accelerating development, improving IQ and adaptive skills compared to those receiving no intervention or alternate diverse standard care treatments.

Most recently, Reichow (2012) presented an overview of the five meta-analyses on EIBI for young children with ASD. He concluded that the collective and accumulating evidence supporting EIBI from meta-analytic studies cannot be dismissed. Reichow's impressive dissection of the investigations of EIBI to date achieves the following assertion:

"Furthermore, the current evidence on the effectiveness of EIBI meets the threshold and criteria for the highest levels of evidence-based treatments across definitions … Collectively, EIBI is the comprehensive treatment model for individuals with ASDs with the greatest amount of empirical support and should be given strong consideration when deciding deciding treatment options for young children with ASDs" (Reichow, 2012, p. 518.)

---

8. Screening for ASD and EIBI provision

It is accepted in the field of autism that there now exists enough evidence to recognise the disorder at a very early age (Feldman et al. 2012; Matson, Boisjoli, Rojahn, & Hess, 2009). While many screening instruments exist for the disorder, the most thoroughly examined of these is the BISCUIT (Matson et al., 2009; Matson, Fodstad, & Mahan, 2009; Matson, Fodstad, Mahan, & Sevin, 2009; Matson, Wilkins, Sevin, et al., 2009; Matson, Wilkins, Sharp, et al., 2009). In addition to providing clinicians with a measure of the very early signs of autism symptomology, the BISCUIT also provides a measure of emotional/behavioural disorders and comorbid psychopathology. We believe that providing EIBI to young infants showing early signs of autism, before the condition is fully manifest, will target core skills by accelerating developmental sequences, halting deteriorating behavioural repertoires, and preventing additional secondary problems. Provision of EIBI at the time when symptoms are initially detected, may in tandem, alter the course of early behavioural and brain development increasing the likelihood that children attain a rate of typical development (Dawson, 2008).

We advocate for the need to screen children for this disorder during routine health and developmental checks. Screening in Ireland is currently haphazard and often depends on a parent showing concern for some area of their child's development. In particular, prevention entails detecting infants at risk before the full diagnostic criteria are present and it has been recognised that early signs may emerge as soon as 9 months in infants with siblings who have ASD (Ozonoff et al. 2010; Zwaigenbaum et al. 2005). Screening these biologically "at risk" children in early infancy should allow greater access to the effective methods demonstrated by EIBI. We strongly believe that the availability of both standardised screening techniques and EIBI provision to such children will impact on a more promising prognosis in the long-term.

9. The benefits of EIBI

There is no doubt that the cost of an intensive and accomplished EIBI program is expensive. For example, cost analysis studies revealed that the average annual cost of an EIBI program in North America to be $33,000 per year with the average duration being three years (Jacobson, Mulick & Green, 1998). However, further analysis of this cost-effectiveness and saving over time has also been provided. For instance, the Autism Society of America reported in 2008 that the cost of lifelong care could be reduced by up to as much as two thirds with early diagnosis and EIBI.

Dillenberger (2011) provides a synopsis of recent cost-benefit analyses showing the savings that can be achieved by implementation of EIBI in autism treatment. She puts forward the following:

1. in Ontario, Canada, an estimated annual CA$ 45 million can be saved if EIBI is made available to all children diagnosed with ASD (see Motiwala et al., 2006);

2. in Texas, USA, a total of US$ 208,500 per child is saved by the education system through the use of EIBI (see Chasson, Harris & Neely (2007);
3. and in Pennsylvania, USA, average savings per child are estimated even higher to range from US$ 274,700 to US$ 282,690 (see also Chasson, Harris & Neely (2007).

Based on these cost-saving analyses increasing change has been shown in policy regarding the role of EIBI in early intervention. For example, the state of Ontario in Canada, has legislated to make EIBI services available for all children diagnosed with ASD (Perry & Condillac, 2003). In the USA, 32 States have passed legislation to ensure that ABA-based interventions are either state-funded or provided through medical insurance companies (Dillenberger, 2011; Market Watch, 2012). It remains to be seen whether government policy in the United Kingdom or Ireland will catch up with that of Canada and the USA and provide government funded EIBI once children are deemed at risk for or indeed presenting with this condition. Interestingly, the use of trained volunteers to deliver EIBI has been shown to produce effective outcomes (Birnbrauer & Leach, 1993) and may be an option for some parents/services to consider when cost is an issue. Many university students who train on third level post-graduate programmes in Applied Behaviour Analysis could make strong contributions in a voluntary capacity, to EIBI in autism treatment, as part of their ongoing accreditation process as Board Certified Behaviour Analysts with the international certification body (Behaviour Analyst Certification Board®). Alternatively providing parents of children with autism with training in behavioural interventions (demonstrated by Sallows and Graupner, 2005) can result in cost-saving and important positive outcomes for children with autism.

10. Controversies related to EIBI efficacy

The published studies outlined in this chapter highlight the possible positive outcomes for young children diagnosed with autism. EIBI continues to be investigated internationally as a treatment intervention for this condition and as a result of these investigations attracts many critics and controversies. In the past, some authors have criticised a behavioural approach to autism intervention with regard to "robotic" teaching and behaviour patterns that lack generalisation to naturalistic settings (Jordan, Jones & Murray, 1998; Shea, 2004) along with the use of negative consequences in acquisition teaching and behaviour reduction (Carr, Robinson & Palumbo, 1990). Others have highlighted the concerns with regard to claims of "recovery"or a "cure" for autism (Offit, 2008). However, the improvements shown over the last decade in EIBI refinement and provision, particularly with regard to training and regulatory protocols with its delivery (Behavior Analyst Certification Board®, 2012) has addressed many of these issues. Indeed, professional training in behaviour analysis and behavioural intervention has never been as well regulated as it is today.

No doubt there are still many issues that continue to require analysis in the EIBI and autism field of research. We would like to draw the reader's attention to a recent publication by Matson and Smith (2008) providing an analysis of the current status of intensive behavioural intervention for young children with autism. We believe that this paper provides an excellent summary of the criticisms provided on EIBI and we will highlight these here. Firstly, many of the studies providing analysis of EIBI outcomes fail to report the severity of ASD across participants and groups. This makes it difficult to decipher which children will show greatest susceptibility to the intervention. Those with greater severity of symptoms may show slower progress or less gains. It has been reported that a milder degree of autism is related to better prognosis (e.g., Bartak & Rutter, 1976) and therefore it is essential that variables at intervention onset include such a measure. Secondly, Matson and Smith (2008) highlight the fact that researchers often do not take into account the additional, co-morbid, problems that present with autism (e.g., ADHD symptoms or anxiety disorders). Psychopathological problems can co-occur with the condition and may exacerbate the challenges and deficits for many children. The impact this can have on treatment susceptibility is underreported and often not addressed in treatment research. For example, only two studies in our review provided outcome measures of co-morbid psychopathology (Birnbrauer & Leach, 1993; Fava, 2011). Matson and Smith (2008) provide a strong argument for the assessment of psychopathology before, during, and after EIBI, to determine ongoing changes in child profiles or to address any required adjustments to the delivery of EIBI (e.g., increasing or decreasing the duration of intervention, removing skills acquisition teaching from artificial environments, less emphasis on massed trial instruction etc.). Perhaps not enough attention has been given to these issues in EIBI research. The young age of onset of EIBI and the intensity of the intervention may have undesired side effects such as anxiety, stress, "burn out" or indeed refusal to participate. Other controversial issues involving EIBI include parent and sibling involvement which can often induce stress and family strain when highly intensive intervention is provided within the family home. The negative side effects of this kind of intensive intervention certainly warrant separate analysis.

Unfortunately, like any professional practice or therapeutic intervention, there will be those who claim to provide EIBI without adhering to the scientific demonstrations of what is, and is not, effective within an intervention protocol. We have heard of anecdotal accounts of the applications of behavioural interventions in autism treatment that are outdated and often lack individualisation. Treatment fidelity is often a major problem in the field and often authors fail to demonstrate or report adherence to effective and current practice in many of the published studies on EIBI. Such problems can lend support to a negative view of the use of EIBI with young children with autism diagnoses.

An analysis of changes in adaptive functioning of young children has become an added focus of EIBI studies in more recent years. Traditionally, studies tended to focus on changes in intellectual and social functioning and language and communication abilities. Some authors have criticised EIBI for overly focusing on cognitive skills with 1:1 teacher/student ratios and a focus on desk-top instruction and intensive "drills" (e.g., Shea, 2004). Increasingly, EIBI curricula and instructional protocols have grown to ensure inclusion of adaptive skills teaching and acquisition of novel skills in natural environments. Studies evaluating outcomes of EIBI have also focused more on adaptive functioning changes as a result of the intervention. In 2002, Eikseth et al. reported greater increases in adaptive functioning in a group of young children who received "eclectic" intervention than those receiving EIBI. Furthermore, Fava et al. (2011) and Strauss et al. (2012) showed that both groups receiving EIBI and "eclectic" intervention showed significant gains in adaptive functioning. Two more recent studies by Eldevik et al.(2012) and Eikseth et al., (2012) reported the opposite findings to Eikseth et al. (2002) in relation to adaptive functioning when comparing both interventions.

Another variable that has been increasingly analysed in early intervention autism research includes parental stress. Interestingly, two comparison studies (Fava et al., 2011; Strauss et al., 2012) showed significant reductions in parental stress for those parents whose children were receiving "eclectic" intervention. The same effect was not shown for parents of children receiving EIBI. This is another important area of analysis particularly in light of the demands that EIBI places on parents and family.

11. Conclusion

EIBI as an approach to autism treatment is one of the most intensively analysed interventions in paediatric clinical psychology (Matson & Smith, 2008).

Substantial objective evidence for EIBI has been demonstrated at an experimental, descriptive and meta-analytic level of analysis (Reichow, 2012). We support the contention of many authors in the field of autism treatment, that EIBI prevails by adhering to a principle of evidence-based practice, incorporating standardised objective measurement of outcomes along with implementation of robust experimental design. This robust demonstration of effectiveness is driving policy change on the international stage and some authors (e.g., Dawson, 2008) suggest that one of the most important goals of investigations in the domains of autism and behaviour analysis research, is to become more effective communicators of scientific findings to the general public/government bodies/advocacy groups/related professionals, not only to harvest their support, but to ensure the dissemination of accurate and effective intervention to so many who require it.

Author details

Olive Healy and Sinéad Lydon

National University of Ireland, Galway

References

[1] Alessandri, M., Thorp, D., Mundy, P., & Tuchman, R. F. (2005). Can we cure autism? From outcome to intervention. *Revista de Neurologia, 40,* S131–S136.

[2] Anderson, S. R., Avery, D. L., DiPietro, E. K., Edwards, G. L., & Christian, W. P. (1987). Intensive home-based early intervention with autistic children. *Education and Treatment of Children, 10,* 353–366.

[3] Autism Treatment Acceleration Act (ATAA). (2010). Summary of the Autism Treatment Acceleration Act of 2009 (ATAA) (S. 819 and H.R. 2413) Retrieved from http://autismtreatmentaccelerationact.org/4.html.

[4] Behavior Analyst Certification Board® (2012). http://www.bacb.com.

[5] Baer, D. M., Wolf, M. M. & Risley, T. R. (1968). Some current dimensions of applied behavior analysis. *Journal of Applied Behavior Analysis, 1,* 91-97.

[6] Baer, D. M., Wolf, M. M. & Risley, T. R. (1987). Some still-current dimensions of applied behavior analysis. *Journal of Applied Behavior Analysis, 20,* 313-317.

[7] Ben-Itzchak, E., Lahat, E., Burgin, R., & Zachor, A. D. (2008). Cognitive, behavior and intervention outcome in young children with autism. *Research in Developmental Disabilities, 29,* 447-458.

[8] Birnbrauer, J. S., & Leach, D. J. (1993). The Murdoch early intervention program after 2 years. *Behaviour Change, 10,* 63-74.

[9] Carr, E.G., Robinson, S., & Palumbo, L.W. (1990). The wrong issue: Aversive versus nonaversive treatment. The right issue: Functional versus non-functional treatment. In A. Repp & N. Singh (Eds.), Perspectives on the use of nonaversive and aversive interventions for persons with developmental disabilities (pp. 361-379). Sycamore, IL: Sycamore Publishing Co.

[10] Chasson, G. S., Harris, G. E., & Neely, W. J. (2007). Cost comparison of early intensive behavioural intervention and special education for children with autism. *Journal of Child and Family Studies, 16,* 401–413.

[11] Cohen, H., Amerine-Dickens, M., & Smith, T. (2006). Early intensive behavioral treatment: Replication of the UCLA model in a community setting. *Developmental and Behavioral Pediatrics, 27,* S145-S155.

[12] Cooper, J. O., Heron, T. E., & Heward, W. L. (2007). *Applied behavior analysis* (2nd ed.). Upper Saddle River, NJ: Prentice Hall.

[13] Dawson, G. (2008). Early behavioral intervention, brain plasticity, and the prevention of autism spectrum disorder. *Development and Psychopathology 20,* 775–803.

[14] Dillenberger, K. (2011). The Emperor's new clothes: Eclecticism in autism treatment. *Research in Autism Spectrum Disorders, 5,* 1119–1128.

[15] Eikeseth, S. (2009). Outcome of comprehensive psycho-educational interventions for young children with autism. *Research in Developmental Disabilities, 30,* 158–178.

[16] Eikeseth, S., Hayward, D., Gale, C., Gitlesen, J. P., & Eldevik, S. (2009). Intensity of supervision and outcome for preschool aged children receiving early and intensive

behavioral interventions: A preliminary study. *Research in Autism Spectrum Disorders, 3*, 67-73. doi: 10.1016/j.rasd.2008.04.003

[17] Eikeseth, S., Klintwall, L., Jahr, E., & Karlsson, P. (2012). Outcome for children with autism receiving early and intensive behavioral intervention in mainstream pre-school and kindergarten settings. *Research in Autism Spectrum Disorders, 6*, 829-835.

[18] Eikeseth, S., Smith, T., Jahr, E., & Eldevik, S. (2002). Intensive behavioral treatment at school for 4- to 7- year old children with autism: A 1-year comparison controlled study. *Behavior Modification, 26*, 49-68.

[19] Eikeseth, S., Smith, T., Jahr, E., & Eldevik, S. (2007). Outcome for children with autism who began intensive behavioral treatment between ages 4 and 7: A comparison controlled study. *Behavior Modification, 31*, 264-278.

[20] Eldevik, S., Hastings, R. P., Hughes, C., Jahr, E., Eikeseth, S., & Cross, S. (2009). Meta-analysis of early intensive behavioral intervention for children with autism. *Journal of Clinical Child and Adolescent Psychology, 38*, 439–450.

[21] Eldevik, S., Eikeseth, S., Jahr, E., & Smith, T. (2006). Effects of low-intensity behavioral treatment for children with autism and mental retardation. *Journal of Autism and Developmental Disorders, 36*, 211-224.

[22] Eldevik, S., Hastings, R. P., Jahr, E., & Hughes, J. C. (2012). Outcomes of behavioral interventions for children with autism in mainstream pre-school settings. *Journal of Autism and Developmental Disorders, 42*, 210-220.

[23] Eldevik, S., Hastings, R. P., Hughes, J. C., Jahr, E., Eikeseth, S., & Cross, S. (2010) Using participant data to extend the evidence base for intensive behavioral intervention for children with autism. *American Journal on Intellectual and Developmental Disabilities, 115*, 381–405.

[24] Fava, L., & Strauss, K. (2011). Cross-setting complementary staff and parent-mediated Early Intensive Behavioral Intervention for young children with autism: Are-search-based comprehensive approach. *Research in Autism Spectrum Disorders, 5*, 512–522.

[25] Fava, L., Strauss, K., Valeri, G., D'Elia, L., Arima, S., & Vicari, S. (2011). The effectiveness of a cross-setting complementary staff- and parent-mediated early intensive behavioral intervention for young children with ASD. *Research in Autism Spectrum Disorders, 5*, 1479-1492.

[26] Feldman M.A., Ward R.A., Savona D., Regehr, K., Parker, K., Hudson, M., Penning, H. & Holden, J.J.A. (2012). Development and initial validation of a parent report measure of the behavioral development of infants at risk for autism spectrum disorders. *Journal of Autism and Developmental Disorders, 42*, 13-22.

[27] Fenske, E. C., Zalenski, S., Krantz, P. J., & McClannahan, L. E. (1985). Age at intervention and treatment outcome for autistic children in a comprehensive intervention program. *Analysis and Intervention in Developmental Disabilities, 5*, 49–58.

[28] Flanagan, H. E., Perry, A., & Freeman, N. L. (2012). Effectiveness of large-scale community-based intensive behavioral intervention: A waitlist comparison study exploring outcomes and predictors. *Research in Autism Spectrum Disorders, 6,* 673-682.

[29] Granpeesheh, D., Tarbox, J., & Dixon, D. R. (2009). Applied behavior analytic interventions for children with autism: A description and review of treatment research. *Annals of Clinical Psychiatry: Official Journal of the American Academy of Clinical Psychiatrist, 21,* 162–173.

[30] Green, G. (1996). Early behavioral intervention for autism: What does research tell us? In C. Maurice, G. Green, & S. Luce (Eds.). *Behavioral intervention for young children with autism: A manual for parents and professionals* (pp. 29- 44). Austin, TX: PRO-ED.

[31] Greer, R.D. (2002). *Designing teaching strategies: an applied behavior analysis systems approach.* Academic Press: Dan Diego, CA.

[32] Greer, R. D., Keohane, D. D. & Healy, O. (2002). Quality and applied behavior analysis. *The Behavior Analyst Today, 3 (2),* 120-132. www.behavior-analyst-today.org.

[33] Gresham, F.M. & MacMillan, D.L. (1998). Early intervention project: Can its claims be substantiated and its effects replicated*? Journal of Autism and Developmental Disorders, 28.* 5-13.

[34] Harris, S. L., Handleman, J. S., Gordon, R., Kristoff, B., & Fuentes, F. (1991). Changes in cognitive and language functioning of preschool children with autism. *Journal of Autism and Developmental Disorders, 21,* 281–290.

[35] Healy, O., Leader, G., & Reed, P. (2009). Applied Behavior Analysis and the Treatment of Autism Spectrum Disorders in the Republic of Ireland. In Leon V. Berhardt (Ed.) Advances in Medicine and Biology, Volume 8. Nova Science Publishers.

[36] Howlin, P. (2010). Evaluating psychological treatments for children with autism-spectrum disorders. *Advances in Psychiatric Treatment, 16,* 133–140.

[37] Hoyson, M., Jamieson, B., & Strain, P. S. (1984). Individualized group instruction of normally developing and autistic-like children: The LEAP Curriculum Model. *Journal of the Division for Early Childhood, 8,* 157-172.

[38] Howard, J. S, Sparkman, C. R., Cohen, H. G., Green, G., & Stanislaw, H. (2005). A comparison of intensive behavior analytic and eclectic treatment for young children with autism. *Research in Developmental Disabilities, 26,* 359-383.

[39] Howlin, P., Magiati, I., & Charman, T. (2009). A systematic review of early intensive behavioural interventions (EIBI) for children with autism. *American Journal on Intellectual and Developmental Disabilities, 114,* 23–41.

[40] Jacobson, J. W., Mulick, J. A., & Green, G. (1998). Cost-benefit estimates for early intensive behavioral intervention for young children with autism: General model and single state case. *Behavioral Interventions, 13,* 201-226.

[41] Jordan R, Jones G, Murray D. (1998). Educational Interventions for Children with Autism: A literature review of recent and current research. School of Education, University of Birmingham, UK.

[42] Keenan, M. & Dillenberger, K. (2011). When all you have is a hammer … : RCTs and hegemony in science. *Research on Autism Spectrum Disorders,* 1-13.

[43] Kelley, E., Naigles, L., & Fein, D. (2010). An in-depth examination of optimal outcome children with a history of autism spectrum disorders. *Research in Autism Spectrum Disorders, 4,* 526-538.

[44] Klintwall, L., & Eikeseth, S. (2012). Number and controllability of reinforcers as predictors of individual outcome for children with autism receiving early and intensive behavioral intervention: A preliminary study. *Research in Autism Spectrum Disorders, 6,* 493-499.

[45] Koegel, Robert L. and Lynn Kern Koegel (2006). *Pivotal Response Treatments for Autism: Communication, Social, and Academic Development.* Baltimore, Md.: Paul H. Brookes.

[46] Kovshoff, H., Hastings, R. P., & Remington, B. (2011). Two-year outcomes for children with autism after the cessation of early intensive behavioral intervention. *Behavior Modification, 35,* 427-450.

[47] Lang, R., O'Reilly, M., Healy, O., Rispoli, M., Lydon, H., Streusand, W., Davis, T., Kang, S., Sigafoos, J., Lancioni, G., Didden, R., & Giesbers, S. (2012). Sensory integration therapy for autism spectrum disorders: A systematic review. *Research in Autism Spectrum Disorders, 6,* 1004-1018

[48] Larsson, E. (2005). Resources for parents. In M. Keenan, M. Henderson, K.P. Kerr, & K. Dillenburger. *Applied behaviour analysis and autism. Building a future togethe*r (pp. 255-287). London: Jessica Kingsley Publishers.

[49] Lovaas, O. I. (1981). *Teaching developmentally disabled children: The me book.* Baltimore: University Park.

[50] Lovaas, O. I. (1987). Behavioral treatment and normal educational and intellectual functioning in young autistic children. *Journal of Consulting and Clinical Psychology, 55,* 3-9.

[51] Lovaas, O. I., Koegel, R., Simmons, J. Q., & Long, J. S. (1973). Some generalization and follow-up measures on autistic children in behavior therapy. *Journal of Applied Behavior Analysis, 6,* 131–166.

[52] Lovaas, O. I., & Smith, T. (1989). A comprehensive behavioraltheory of autistic children: Paradigm for research andtreatment. Journal of Behavior Therapy and Experimental Psychiatry, 20, 17–29.

[53] Love, J. R., Carr, J. E., Almason, S. M., & Petursdottir, A. I. (2009). Early and intensive behavioral intervention for autism: A survey of clinical practices. *Research in Autism Spectrum Disorders, 3,* 421-428.

[54] Magiati, I., Charman, T., & Howlin, P. (2007). A two-year prospective follow-up study of community-based early intensive behavioural intervention and specialist nursery provision for children with autism spectrum disorders. *Journal of Child Psychology and Psychiatry, 48,* 803-812.

[55] Magiati, I., & Howlin, P. (2001). Monitoring the progress of preschool children with autism enrolled in early intervention programmers. *Autism, 5,* 399–406.

[56] Market Watch (2012). http://www.marketwatch.com/story/department-of-defense-and-tri-care-ordered-to-provide-applied-behavioral-therapy-to-autistic-children-of-military-dependents-2012-07-26.

[57] Makrygianni, M. K., & Reed, P. (2010). A meta-analytic review of the effectiveness of behavioural early intervention programs for children with autism spectrum disorders. *Research in Autism Spectrum Disorders, 4,* 577–593.

[58] Matson, J. L. Benavidez, D. A., Compton, L. S., Paclawskyj, T. R., & Baglio, C. S. (1996). Behavioral treatment for autistic persons: A review of research from 1980 to the present. *Research in Developmental Disabilities, 17,* 433–466.

[59] Matson, J. L., Boisjoli, J., Rojahn, J., & Hess, J. (2009). A factor analysis of challenging behaviors assessed with the Baby and Infant Screen for Children with aUtIsm Traits (BISCUIT-Part 3). *Research in Autism Spectrum Disorders, 3,* 714–722.

[60] Matson, J. L., Fodstad, J. C., & Mahan, S. (2009). Cutoffs, norms, and patterns of comorbid difficulties in children with developmental disabilities on the Baby Infant Screen for Children with aUtIsm Traits (BISCUIT-Part 2). *Research in Developmental Disabilities, 30,* 1221–1228.

[61] Matson, J. L., Fodstad, J. C., Mahan, S., & Sevin, J. A. (2009). Cutoffs, norms, and patterns of comorbid difficulties in children with ASD on the Baby Infant Screen for Children with aUtIsm Traits (BISCUIT-Part 2). *Research in Autism Spectrum Disorders, 3,* 977–988.

[62] Matson, J. L., Wilkins, J., Sevin, J. A., Knight, C., Boisjoli, J. A., & Sharp, B. (2009). Reliability and item content of the Baby and Infant Screen for Children with aUtIsm Traits (BISCUIT): Part 1–3. *Research in Autism Spectrum Disorders, 3,* 336–344.

[63] Matson, J. L., & Smith, K. R. M. (2008). Current status of intensive behavioral interventions for young children with autism and PDD-NOS. *Research in Autism Spectrum Disorders, 2,* 60–74.

[64] Matson, J.L., Tureck, K., Turygin, N., Beighley, J., Rieske, R. (2012). Trends and topics in Early Intensive Behavioral Interventions for toddlers with autism. *Research in Autism Spectrum Disorders, 6,* 1412–1417.

[65] McEachin, J. J., Smith, T., & Lovaas, O. I. (1993). Long-term outcome for children with autism who received early intensive behavioral treatment. *American Journal on Mental Retardation, 97,* 359–391.

[66] McGarrell, M., Healy, O., Leader, G., O'Connor, J., & Kenny, N. (2009). Six reports of children with autism spectrum disorder following intensive behavioural interventions using the Preschool Inventory of Repertoires for Kindergarten (PIRRK®). *Research in Autism Spectrum Disorders, 3,* 767–782.

[67] Metz, Mulick, J., and Butter, E. (2005). Autism: A late-20th-century fad magnet. In J. W. Jacobson, R. M. Foxx, and J. A. Mulick (Eds.), *Controversial therapies for developmental disabilities: Fad, fashion, and science in professional practice.* Mahwah, New Jersey: Lawrence Erlbaum Associates.

[68] Motiwala, S. S., Gupta, S., Lilly, M. B., Ungar, W. J., & Coyte, P. C. (2006). The cost-effectiveness of expanding intensive behavioural intervention to all autistic children in Ontario. *Health Policy, 1,* 135–151.

[69] Mudford, O., et al., (2009). Technical review of published research on applied behaviour analysis interventions for people with autism spectrum disorders: Auckland Uniservices Ltd. Wellington, New Zealand: Ministry of Education.

[70] Mulloy, A., Lang, R., O'Reilly, M., Sigafoos, J., Lancioni, G., & Rispoli, M. (2010). Gluten-free and casein-free diets in the treatment of autism spectrum disorders: A systematic review. *Research in Autism Spectrum Disorders, 4,* 328-339.

[71] Mundy, P., Sullivan, L., & Mastergeorge, A. (2009). A parallel and distributed-processing model of joint attention, social cognition and autism. Autism research, 2, 2–21.

[72] Offit, Paul (2008). *Autism's False Prophets: Bad Science, Risky Medicine, and the Search for a Cure.* Columbia University Press: New York.

[73] Ozonoff, S., Iosif, A.-M., Baguio, F., Cook, I. C., Hill, M. M., Hutman, T., et al. (2010). A prospective study of the emergence of early behavioral signs of autism. *Journal of the American Academy of Child & Adolescent Psychiatry, 49(3),* 258–268.

[74] Perry, A., & Condillac, R. (2003). *Evidence-based practices for children and adolescents with autism spectrum disorders: Review of the literature and practice guide.* Ontario, Canada: Children's Mental Health Ontario.

[75] Perry, A., Cummings, A., Geier, J. D., Freeman, N. L., Hughes, S., Managhan, T., et al. (2011). Predictors of outcome for children receiving intensive behavioral intervention in a large community-based program. *Research in Autism Spectrum Disorders, 5,* 592–603.

[76] Peters-Scheffer, N., Didden, R., Korzilius, H., & Matson, J. (2012). Cost comparison of early intensive behavioral intervention and treatment as usual for children with autism spectrum disorder in the Netherlands. *Research in Developmental Disabilities, 33,* 1763-1772.

[77] Reed, P., Osborne, L. A., & Corness, M. (2007a). Brief report: Relative effectiveness of different home-based behavioral approaches to early teach intervention. *Journal of Autism and Developmental Disorders, 37,* 1815-1821.

[78] Reed, P., Osborne, L. A., & Corness, M. (2007b). The real-world effectiveness of early teaching interventions for children with autism spectrum disorder. *Exceptional Children, 73,* 417-433.

[79] Reichow, B. (2012). Overview of Meta-Analyses on Early Intensive Behavioral Intervention for Young Children with Autism Spectrum Disorders. *Journal of Autism and Developmental Disorders, 42,* 512–520.

[80] Reichow, B., & Wolery, M. (2009). Comprehensive synthesis of early intensive behavioral interventions for young children with autism based on the UCLA Young Autism Project model. *Journal of Autism and Developmental Disorders, 39,* 23–41.

[81] Remington, B., Hastings, R. P., Kovshoff, H., degli Espinosa, F., Jahr, E., Brown, T. & Ward, N. (2007). Early intensive behavioral intervention: Outcomes for children with autism and their parents after two years. *American Journal on Mental Retardation, 112,* 418-438.

[82] Rogers, S. J., & Vismara, L. A. (2008). Evidence-based comprehensive treatments for early autism. *Journal of Clinical Child and Adolescent Psychology, 37,* 8–38.

[83] Sallows, G. O., & Graupner, T. D. (2005). Intensive behavioral treatment for children with autism: Four-year outcome and predictors. *American Journal on Mental Retardation, 110,* 417-438.

[84] Schopler, E., Short, A., & Mesibov, G. (1989). Relation of behavioral treatment to normal functioning: Comment on Lovaas. Journal of Consulting and Clinical Psychology, 57, 162-164.

[85] Sheinkopf, S. J., & Siegel, B. (1998). Home-baseed behavioral treatment of young children with autism. *Journal of Autism and Developmental Disorders, 28,* 15-23.

[86] Schreibman, L. (2000). Intensive behavioral/psychoeducational treatments for autism: Research needs and future directions. *Journal of Autism and Developmental Disorders, 30,* 373–378.

[87] Shea, V. (2004). A perspective on the research literature related to early intensive behavioral intervention (Lovaas) for young children with autism. *Autism, 8,* 349–367.

[88] Smith, T. (1999). Outcome of early intervention for children with autism. *Clinical Psychology: Science and Practice, 6,* 33–49.

[89] Smith, T., Eikeseth, S., Klevstrand, M., & Lovaas, O. I. (1997). Intensive behavioral treatment for preschoolers with severe mental retardation and pervasive developmental disorder. *American Journal on Mental Retardation, 102,* 238-249.

[90] Smith, T., Eikeseth, S., Sallows, G. O., & Graupner, T. D. (2010). Efficacy of applied behavior analysis in autism. *The Journal of Pediatrics, 155,* 151–152.

[91] *Smith, T., Groen, A. D., & Wynn, J. W. (2000). Randomized trial of intensive early intervention for children with pervasive developmental disorder. *American Journal on Mental Retardation, 105*, 269-285.

[92] Spreckley, M., & Boyd, R. (2009). Efficacy of applied behavioral intervention in preschool children with autism for improving cognitive, language, and adaptive behavior: A systematic review and meta-analysis. *The Journal of Pediatrics, 154*, 338–344.

[93] Steege, M. W., Mace, C., Perry, L., & Longenecker, H. (2007). Applied behavior analysis: Beyond discrete trial teaching. *Psychology in the Schools, 44*, 91–99.

[94] Strauss, K., Vicari, S., Valeri, G., D'Elia, L., Arima, S., & Fava, L. (2012). Parent inclusion in early intensive behavioral intervention: The influence of parental stress, parent treatment fidelity and parent-mediated generalization of behavior targets on child outcomes. *Research in Developmental Disabilities, 33*, 688-703.

[95] Sundberg, M. L., & Michael, J. (2001). The value of Skinner's analysis of verbal behavior for teaching children with autism. *Behavior Modification*, 25, 698-724.

[96] Symes, M. D., Remington, B., & Brown, T. (2006). Early intensive intervention for children with autism: Therapists' perspective on achieving procedural fidelity. *Research in Developmental Disabilities, 27*, 30–42.

[97] Virue´s-Ortega, J. (2010). Applied behavior analytic intervention for autism in early childhood: Meta-analysis, meta-regression and dose-response meta-analysis of multiple outcomes. *Clinical Psychology Review, 30*, 387–399.

[98] Zwaigenbaum, L., Bryson, S., Rogers, T., Roberts, W., Brian, J., & Szatmari, P. (2005). Behavioral manifestations of autism in the first year of life. International *Journal of Developmental Neuroscience, 23*, 143–152.

Chapter 3

Clinical Approach in Autism: Management and Treatment

Rudimar Riesgo, Carmem Gottfried and Michele Becker

Additional information is available at the end of the chapter

1. Introduction

The terms Autism and ASD (Autism Spectrum Disorders) can be interchangeable in the clinical setting, and have been used to describe one of the most intriguing neurobehavioral syndromes, that include the so-called "triad of Wing": problems in communication, social skills, and restrict repertoire of interests. However, it is somewhat difficult to precisely define autism, because of the imprecise boundaries between different kinds of ASD as well as the fact that there is no biological marker to date (Gottfried and Riesgo 2011).

By definition, in autism the social deficits are characterized by lack of interest in spontaneously sharing feelings, different levels of communication deficits, difficulties in imaginative plays, restrictive repertoire of interests, non-functional routine fixations, as well as stereotypies and other motor alterations, such as flapping with hands, circular movements and others (Nikolov, Jonker, and Scahill 2006; Gadia, Tuchman, and Rotta 2004).

While the criteria of the DSM-V (Diagnostic and Statistical Manual of Mental Disorders – Fifth Edition) are not yet published, we still have to use the "older version". According with the DSM–IV criteria, there are five clinical situations that could be encompassed by the term "PDD" (Pervasive Developmental Disorders) or "ASD" (Autism Spectrum Disorders) with the same meaning of PDD or autism (Association 2002).

Although it will change in the near future, the five current clinical ASD diagnosis admitted by DSM-IV-TR (Gadia et al., 2004) are: a) Autistic Disorder; b) Asperger Disorder (AD); c) Rett Disorder; d) Childhood Disintegrative Disorder; e) PDD-NOS (Pervasive Developmental Disorder – Not Otherwise Specified).

According with DSM-IV-TR, and in agreement with previous epidemiological data, our group found that the most prevalent ASD is the PDD-NOS, followed by Autistic Disorder, and then by Asperger Disorder. Accordingly, the Rett Disorder and the Childhood Disintegrative Disorder for sure are less frequently seen in the clinical practice (Longo et al. 2009).

The increasing levels of prevalence in ASD probably is due to several reasons, such as the changes in diagnostic criteria, the high level of awareness, the underestimation of former data, the massive information exchange regarding ASD, the public strategies, etc. The first description of autism was made by Hans Asperger, in 1938. In 1943, when Leo Kanner described a sample with 11 children, autism was a rare condition affecting not more than 4 in 10.000 children (Kanner 1943).

However, childhood autism is much more frequent and is identified in at least one in each 100 children nowadays. For instance, a recent paper describes prevalence of 2.6% of ASD in children aging from seven to twelve years of age (Kim et al. 2011).

Autism and ASD certainly have different kinds of approaches. These neurobehavioral syndromes can be addressed, for example, both from the clinical and from the experimental field. To our knowledge, at least in the academic environment, the best approach could be the translational type because it made us able to rapidly build a bridge between the experimental and the clinical field (Gottfried and Riesgo 2011).

Obviously, the earlier results usually came from the experimental research for several reasons. In general, the time spent in each one experiment can be shorter compared to clinical research; the environmental variables can be in part controlled, etc. By the other side, clinical research can be more time consuming and potentially more complicated to be performed. There is no doubt that both approaches are not mutually exclusive. Actually they are complementary.

Strictly speaking from the clinical perspective in autism, we can divide the clinical approach into two basic and complementary issues. The first one is the general management, including the confirmation of the correct diagnosis, the determination of the intensity of the compromise, and the evaluation of intensity level of eventual core behavioral symptoms. The last one encompasses several treatment options, which includes psychopharmacotherapy and different types of non-medical treatments.

As the first cases of autism were described in the early 40's, now we have adults with ASD. That is the reason to keep in mind how ASD symptoms usually change during lifetime. As time pass, different symptoms change differently and it is crucial to clinicians to know these differences.

In this context, the present chapter aimed to review (i) the general management of ASD from the clinical perspective; (ii) the lifetime changes in ASD symptoms; and (iii) the evidence-based treatment options.

2. General management of ASD from the clinical perspective

The general management of ASD from the clinical perspective encompasses both interventions in the family/environment as well as interventions addressed to the patient. Ideally, after diagnosis confirmation, the best initial approach could be done by an interdisciplinary team including professionals coming from medicine, psychology and social sciences.

Obviously, before initiating any kind of intervention, several steps must be done as follows. First of all, the final diagnosis must be confirmed by a careful anamnesis as well double-checked using the DSM-IV criteria as well as a reliable clinical instrument such as Autism Diagnosis Interview-Revised (ADI-R) (Becker et al. 2012). The ADI-R is frequently used as a gold standard instrument for publication purposes, but it is problematic in the clinical practice for several reasons, such as it can miss same ASD cases as well as it need at least two hours to be completed. Then, the intensity of the ASD could be defined both from the clinical perspective and by one instrument such as CARS (Pereira, Riesgo, and Wagner 2008). Another critical issue is to delimitate if there is any associated mental disability and its degree of intensity. As clinicians, we know the prognostic importance of an unaffected intelligence in ASD patients.

The second step includes the definition of the parent's doubts, fears, and degree of awareness. Usually, after diagnosis confirmation, parents became stressed. Not infrequently they go to internet in order to search every kind of available information regarding autism. Because some information coming from internet can be inaccurate, at this point, it is very important to clarify which are the evidence-based types of therapies to date.

The third step could be the delimitation of environmental variables that needs to be addressed, starting from the home and family. Neighborhood and school needs to be evaluated both in terms of potential stressors and also because they can facilitates choosing a given type of therapy on an individual basis.

The next step is done by the identification of the target behaviors needing treatment. After core symptoms definition in each case, the different professional specialties that need to be involved are selected. In general, the team includes a physician specialized in ASD patients as well as one speech therapist and others professionals arising from health care and/or education with experience in children with ASD.

3. How ASD symptoms change during lifetime

All professionals who treat children and adolescents, both coming from health care as well as from education must know how behaviors can normally change during the normal neuropsychological development. In other words: there is an ontogenetic evolution on each one of the behavioral manifestations in the normally developed children.

For example: in terms of gender versus behavior, usually hyperactivity is more prevalent in normal boys when compared with normal girls. The humor control, the language skills and the social competence usually improves in normally developed children as long as time passes. Usually, normal girls tend to improve faster their language skills and their social competence when compared with normal boys. This knowledge is crucial to identify how different behavioral symptoms change during lifetime in ASD patients.

When the issue is childhood autism symptoms, there are no major problems in terms of information, because of most of the available publications are directed to pediatric patients. As a consequence, adult ASD symptoms are less frequently accessed in the available literature.

Researchers had noted that the prevalence of adult ASD may be underestimating and most of these patients reach adulthood without any diagnosis or treatment. This is especially true to patients with Asperger. (Szatmari et al. 1995; Arora et al. 2011).

More recently, an increasing interest is observed in prevalence and clinical presentation of ASD in adults. The few available prospective studies indicate a diagnostic stability through life (Billstedt, Gillberg, and Gillberg 2005), and near of 80% of individuals with ASD diagnosed in childhood continues to present scores within this spectrum during adolescence and adulthood (Rutter, Greenfeld, and Lockyer 1967).

It is important to mention the difficulties in making diagnosis of ASD in adult patients, because many of them have no information regarding their first years of life. If the diagnosis of ASD is hard to be made in adults, then the prognosis is equally affected. The prognostic studies in adults with ASD had includes patients with very different levels of cognitive, linguistic, social, and behavioral functioning (Howlin et al. 2004). Additionally, most of available the prognostic studies in adult ASD use small samples, which make impossible to obtain definitive conclusions.

Where searching literature regarding how ASD symptoms change during lifetime, a paucity of published information is promptly identified. Although the lack of publications, at least two different timelines could be identified in ASD patients: a) how ASD core symptoms change as time pass; b) how ASD-associated symptoms change with time.

3.1. How ASD core symptoms change during lifetime

The three core symptoms of ASD, the so-called "triad of Wing" are the following: social deficits, communication deficits, and restrict and repetitive behavior.

The social deficits persist as an important problem in adolescence and adult age and usually are accessed by the Autism Diagnostic Interview (ADI) and also by the Vineland Adaptive Behavior Scale (VABS). Our group translated into Brazilian Portuguese the ADI-R, considered the "gold-standard" in autism diagnosis and is extremely useful identifying social deficits (Becker et al. 2012). One study found that only 16.7% of adults with autism presented high scores in social domain of VABS. Additionally, more than half of patients had no social contact at all and one third showed strange social contact (Howlin, Mawhood, and Rutter 2000). In general, social deficits do not improve significantly as time pass.

The communication skills tend to improve. As a group, ASD patients tend to keep almost unchanged the idiosyncratic use of language as well as the inappropriate patterns of communication in adulthood. More recent research had shown that more than half of ASD patients present language below the level of ten years of age, when adults. When comparing ASD versus AD patients with similar age and cognition, it is identified a slight superiority in language skills in the AD patient group (Mawhood, Howlin, and Rutter 2000; Howlin et al. 2004).

The restrictive repertoire of activities and interests do not change in intensity as long as time passes, but certainly the type of interest do change during lifetime. Only few studies address the restrictive repertoire of interests. According with Rutter and colleagues (1967), in a cohort study, although some improvement was identified, all of patients with repetitive behaviors during infancy continued presenting it 10 years later, with a trend to increasing frequency and intensity of such symptoms (Rutter, Greenfeld, and Lockyer 1967). Subsequent research showed that near of 90% of adolescents and adults with autism persisted with restrictive repertoire of activities and interests (Seltzer et al. 2003; Howlin et al. 2004).

Another recurrent preoccupation in ASD follow up is regarding the Intellectual Quotient (IQ). Although some studies revealed lifelong IQ stability, it seem to have a performance IQ decline and a verbal IQ increase as time pass. In reality, there is a paucity of studies regarding IQ changes lifelong in ASD patients. In patients with verbal and performance IQ above 70, these changes seem to be less intense (Howlin et al. 2004).

Core symptom	In adolescence	In adulthood
Social deficits	Persistence of social deficits. A discrete improvement can occur	Persistence of social deficits. A discrete improvement can occur
Communication deficits	Can improve, but some deficits persists	Can improve, but some deficits persists
Restrict repetitive behavior	Increase in frequency and complexity	Persists in 90%. Uncommon concerns and complex stereotypies can decrease. The focus of interests can vary

Table 1. How ASD core symptoms change during lifetime.

3.2. How ASD-associated symptoms change with time

There are few epidemiologic studies of the ASD-associated comorbidities changes as time pass. Consequently, to date any estimate need to be taken with caution.

In general, the comorbidities found in classic autism are different from the identified in Asperger patients, which is probably associated with cognition. As a result, classic autism is more associated to violent behavior, and psychosis. By the other side, Asperger disorder can be more linked to anxiety and/or depression.

The more prevalent psychiatric diagnosis in ASD patients is depression that seems to become more intense with age and frequently associated with anxiety (Howlin, Mawhood, and Rutter 2000). In our experience, the dyad depression/anxiety is more frequent in intelligence-preserved ASD patients, such as those with Asperger disorder. Additionally, anxiety seems to increase in stress situations and also during lifetime (Gottfried and Riesgo 2011). Because of their ability to identify their own difficulties (Cederlund, Hagberg, and Gillberg 2010), patients with Asperger are more prone to became depressed.

The second more frequent psychiatric disorder in ASD patients is probably bipolar disorder (Howlin, Mawhood, and Rutter 2000). Young ASD children experience more difficulties in mood stabilization. In addition, mood's changes occur more rapidly in children when compared with adults. As a result, in very young ASD children the humor can change almost instantaneously.

The prevalence of bipolar disorders as a whole can reach up to 33% in ASD patients (Abramson et al. 1992). Obsessive and compulsive symptoms are frequently identified in ASD, although is difficult to distinguish the pure obsessive-compulsive disorder from bizarre concerns common in patients with autism (Howlin, Mawhood, and Rutter 2000).

Adults with Asperger disorder can experience occasional episodes of psychosis, such as persecutory ideas, auditory hallucinations, paranoid idea or delusional thoughts. But schizophrenia is not common and must remain as a differential diagnosis (Howlin, Mawhood, and Rutter 2000). The abovementioned episodes of psychosis can be identified in up to 15% of Asperger patients after adolescence (Hofvander et al. 2009).

Hyperactivity is a frequent symptom in children with ASD, is more prevalent in boys than in girls, and can decrease as time passes. Although the concomitant aggressiveness itself usually decrease with aging, the consequences of aggressiveness can be worse with age increasing in patients with autism because of their increase of muscle strength. An overlap between ADHD and ASD is relatively common in childhood, but this association is rarely described in manuscripts with ASD adults (Stahlberg et al. 2004).

3.3. Prognosis for ASD patients in adulthood

Although there are no doubts regarding a substantial improvement in the management of autism in the last three decades, unfortunately even nowadays a minority of adults with autism is able to work, to live independently, as well to develop appropriate social skills. Most of these patients still live with their parents or other caregivers (Howlin et al. 2004).

It is known by far that the most important prognostic value is defined by the cognitive functioning in childhood. In this sense, the clinical problem eventually is to access intelligence in non-verbal ASD children. According with literature, children with autism and IQ above 70 had better global prognosis in adulthood (Howlin et al. 2004).

The ability to acquire functional language until the age of six years is also another prognostic landmark (Howlin et al. 2004). Better language and more preserved cognition are the two probably reasons to explain the best prognosis in Asperger disorder when compared with classical forms of autism.

4. Psychopharmacological treatment of ASD patients

Since to date there is no specific medication developed to autism itself, the psychopharmacologic approach is addressed to some core symptoms, such as hyperactivity, anxiety, depression, etc. Actually, medication is frequently required to decrease the "noise" surrounding autism, including a wide range of maladaptive behaviors and/or associated problems (Benvenuto et al. 2012). To our knowledge, psychopharmacotherapy can eventually improve adhesion to non-medical treatment of ASD patients (Gottfried and Riesgo 2011).

In our experience, we usually identify 2-5 ASD associated symptoms and/or diagnosis, including epilepsy. We have found disruptive behavior more frequently in ASD patients with cognitive impairment, as well as symptoms related with depression and/or anxiety in preserved intelligence ASD children (Gottfried and Riesgo 2011). Other related symptoms are: aggression, self-injury, impulsivity, decreased attention, anxiety, depression, and sleep disruption, among others.

Because ASD are chronic and markedly impairing situations in many cases, there is justifiably a high desire for effective treatments. By the other side, it is important to mention that there is a paucity of well conducted evidence-based studies of medications used in ASD patients. Not infrequently, this desire leads to premature enthusiasm for agents and interventions that appear promising in early reports but later do not withstand the rigor of randomized controlled trial (RTC).

Another critical issue is the co-occurrence of epilepsy in ASD patients which is almost twenty times more frequent when ASD patients are compared with children with typical development. The management of combined epilepsy can represent a challenge for clinicians. Several anti-epileptic drugs can determine an exacerbation of behavioral symptoms, and some psychotropic medications used in ASD patients may lower the seizure threshold (Benvenuto et al. 2012). In our experience, risperidone can be safely used up to 3mg/Kg/day, and higher doses can lead to seizures in susceptible patients. That is the reason why we prefer to perform an electroencephalogram before using psychoactive drugs in ASD children (Gottfried and Riesgo 2011). Therefore, it's mandatory to search a treatment strategy with the minor negative impact on this subgroup of patients

It should be noted that most psychotropic use in ASD is actually off-label, as currently there are only two medications approved for use in ASD children by the FDA (Food and Drug Administration). These drugs are risperidone and aripiprazole, which are effective to associated behaviors, but not to autism itself. The general principles for the pharmacotherapy in ASD are similar to the used in other neuropsychiatric conditions (Weinssman and Bridgemohan 2012).

In summary, the use of psychotropic medications, alone or in combination, should follow some guidelines, such as: be focused on specific targets, be used at the minimum effective dosage, as well as be used for short period of time (Benvenuto et al. 2012). Ideally, medications should be initiated only after behavioral and educational interventions are in place.

4.1. Disruptive behaviors

Disruptive behaviors in ASD children may include irritability, aggression, explosive outbursts (tantrums), and/or self-injury. These symptoms can be identified in almost two thirds of ASD patients and certainly have the biggest impact on the care of affected individuals, as well as marked distress for their families (Benvenuto et al. 2012; Kanne and Mazurek 2011). Although behavioral and environmental approaches are recommended as the initial treatment, more severe or even dangerous behaviors usually result in requests for urgent pharmacologic intervention (Kaplan and McCracken 2012; Weinssman and Bridgemohan 2012). In our experience, this type of symptoms is more frequently found in intelligence disabled ASD patients (Gottfried and Riesgo 2011).

In the past, conventional neuroleptic agents such as haloperidol have been used in disruptive behaviors of autistic patients (Benvenuto et al. 2012; Miral et al. 2008; Kaplan and McCracken 2012). Our group showed that risperidone is superior when compared with haloperidol in one experimental research using hippocampal cells (Quincozes-Santos et al. 2010). Additionally, in the clinical research, at least one study proved that risperidone is more effective than haloperidol in ASD patients (Miral et al. 2008). There are two RTC suggesting that haloperidol is effective in disruptive behaviors of ASD children (Campbell et al. 1982; Miral et al. 2008), but sedation and other side effects including dyskinesia and extrapyramidal symptoms limits its use (Weinssman and Bridgemohan 2012).

As a result, to date atypical antipsychotic seem to be more helpful in treatment of disruptive behaviors. Currently, risperidone and aripiprazole are the only second-generation antipsychotic drugs that have shown to decrease disruptive behaviors in large-scale, controlled, double-blind studies (Benvenuto et al. 2012; Kaplan and McCracken 2012; Weinssman and Bridgemohan 2012).

Before the approval by FDA in 2006, risperidone was carefully studied by the NIMH Research Units on Pediatric Psychopharmacology (RUPP) Autism Network. A multiphasic trial comparing risperidone with placebo was performed by RUPP for the treatment of aggressive behaviors in patients aged 5 to 17 years with ASD. There was an initial double-blind, 8-week RCT study (McCracken et al. 2002).

The studies found that risperidone, in mean doses of 2,08mg/d, was effective for reducing moderate to severe tantrums, aggression, and self-injurious behavior in children with autism. There wasn't evidence of side effects such as dyskinesia or dystonia. However, the observed weight gain of 5,6kg for the risperidone group was more than twice the expected weight gain over a 6-month period (McCracken et al. 2002; Kaplan and McCracken 2012).

Risperidone was approved by the FDA in 2006 for the treatment of disruptive symptoms in children and adolescents aged from 5 to 16 years with autism, with a maximum recommended dose of 3 mg/d. In our experience, risperidone was initially used in dose up to 6 mg/d. As time pass, we noted that if no response was obtained with 3mg/d, no more increments were useful. Coincidentally, this daily regimen seems to be the seizure threshold in susceptible patients (Gottfried and Riesgo 2011).

Aripiprazole was approved by the FDA for the treatment of disruptive behavior in ASD patients aged 6 to 17 years in 2009. Two large controlled studies documented the short-term efficacy of aripiprazole at 5, 10 or 15 mg/d for severe aggression and irritability in young subjects with autistic disorder. The most commonly reported adverse events were drowsiness and weight gain, with extrapyramidal symptoms mostly in the fixed-dose study, but these events rarely led to treatment discontinuation (Marcus et al. 2009; Owen et al. 2009). Aripiprazole dosing and response can vary considerably; the usual recommended clinical dose for maintenance is between 5 and 15 mg/d (Kaplan and McCracken 2012).

Other atypical antipsychotics lack large-scale controlled studies. Small open-label reports suggest variable benefits of olanzapine (Potenza et al. 1999), clozapine (Beherec et al. 2011), and ziprasidone (Malone et al. 2007), which have possible support, versus quetiapine, which has not appeared to be beneficial. Other medications of different classes have been used, such as alpha-2 agonists, mood stabilizers, beta blockers, SSRI (selective serotonin reuptake inhibitors), all of them without evidence-based studies of efficacy in disruptive behavior to date (Weinssman and Bridgemohan 2012).

Probably due the co-occurrence of epilepsy in ASD, the use of some antiepileptic drugs has been used in the management of maladaptive behaviors (Gottfried and Riesgo 2011). Divalproex sodium has been demonstrated to be efficient not only in decreasing irritability/aggression, but also in improving of repetitive behaviors, social relatedness and mood instability (Hollander et al. 2006; Hollander et al. 2010).

Adjunctive topiramate therapies can decrease irritability, hyperactivity and inattention (Hardan, Jou, and Handen 2004; Mazzone and Ruta 2006). Moreover, the combination of topiramate with risperidone has been proved superior to risperidone monotherapy in reducing irritability and severe disruptive symptoms (Rezaei et al. 2010). In our experience, this specific combination would be helpful in preventing or at least decreasing the weight gain due to risperidone usage in ASD patients.

Although preliminary data of open-label studies showed that levetiracetam may reduce hyperactivity, impulsivity, mood instability and aggression in autistic children, a RCT suggest that levetiracetam does not improve behavioral disturbances of ASD (Weinssman and Bridgemohan 2012), as well lamotrigine (Belsito et al. 2001).

4.2. Hyperactivity and inattention symptoms

These symptoms are frequently identified in ASD patients. Inattention, hyperactivity and impulsivity may be related to comorbid ADHD (attention deficit hyperactivity disorder) and/or to baseline anxiety of these children (Murray 2010; Rommelse et al. 2010; Benvenuto et al. 2012) Weinssman & Bridgemohan, 2012). It is known that children with ASD and ADHD have more clinical impairments than children with ASD alone (Gadow, DeVincent, and Pomeroy 2006; Kaplan and McCracken 2012).

The potentially useful drugs for inattention and hyperactivity in ASD could be stimulants, alpha-2 adrenergic agonists, atypical antipsychotics as well as anticonvulsant mood stabilizers. To date, there is strong evidence that both stimulants and risperidone are effective for hyperactivity. If the inattention and/or hyperactivity behaviors are due to anxiety, SSRI may be a useful choice (Weinssman and Bridgemohan 2012).

Psychoestimulants and other medications used in typically developing children with ADHD have been evaluated as a therapeutic option for treatment of ADHD symptoms in patients with ASD. The largest trial undertaken by RUPP Autism Network has demonstrated that methylphenidate (MPH) was reasonably efficacious in patient with both ASD and ADHD (RUPP 2005). Convergent evidence from different studies confirms a positive effect on social behaviors (joint attention, response to bids for joint attention, self-regulation, and regulated affective sate), hyperactivity, inattention and impulsiveness (Di Martino et al. 2004; Jahromi et al. 2009). However, response rate to MPH is lower in ASD children compared with children with ADHD without ASD (Weinssman and Bridgemohan 2012). In ASD children, MPH should be started at the lowest dosage ant titrated slowly because of these patients are more prone to experience side effects.

As the same observed with MPH, atomoxetine has initially demonstrated a lower efficacy in ASD patients with ADHD than in ADHD children without autism (Posey et al. 2007; Charnsil 2011). Nevertheless, more recent studies showed significant reductions in ADHD symptoms in high-functioning ASD boys (Zeiner, Gjevik, and Weidle 2011).

Regarding the use of antipsychotic drugs in inattentive/hyperactive ASD patients, secondary analyses from large RTCs demonstrated that risperidone and aripiprazole are associated with large reduction of hyperactivity in children with ASD (McCracken et al. 2002; Owen et al. 2009; Weinssman and Bridgemohan 2012).

Despite the small number of RCT, another option is the use of alpha-2 agonists drugs in ASD children with inattention, hyperactivity, and impulsivity. The use of guanfacine in autistic children has showed modest improvement in the domains of hyperactivity, inattention, insomnia, and tics (Scahill et al. 2006; Handen, Sahl, and Hardan 2008; Weinssman and Bridgemohan 2012). Clonidine is effective in reducing sleep disorders of children with ASD, with a consequent daily improvement of attention deficits, hyperactivity, mood instability and aggressiveness (Jaselskis et al. 1992; Ming et al. 2008). However, only two RCT have been conducted for this class of agent (Weinssman and Bridgemohan 2012).

4.3. Stereotypy and repetitive behaviors

One of the core symptoms in ASD children is perseverative or repetitive behaviors usually associated with difficulties in change interests, which can interfere in the quality of life of patients and parents. Stereotypies and repetitive behaviors are not unique to ASD and can be found in other developmental disorders, although clinicians and researchers agree that these tend to be more frequent in ASD (Kaplan & McCracken, 2012; Leekam et al., 2011). By the other hand, difficulties in changing interests, in the context of a developmental disorder, is one of the hallmarks of autism.

Before use of medication, behavioral therapies should be performed. In our experience, poor cognitive performance can be one of the limitations to behavioral therapy. If the child is mentally disabled, the non-medical approach can be unsuccessful. In this situation, when these symptoms are intense enough to cause impairments to academic performance and/or interpersonal relationships, pharmacologic treatment is often considered.

Because of the similarity of this cluster of autistic symptoms to anxiety as well as other serotonin-related disorders such as obsessive compulsive disorder has led clinicians to use and researchers to investigate the efficacy of SSRI in the treatment of repetitive behaviors and rigidity. Other possibilities in terms of medication include clomipramine, atypical antipsychotics and valproate (Weinssman & Bridgemohan, 2012).

To date, although the lack of high quality evidence that SSRI are effective to stereotypy and repetitive behaviors, we still use this class of medication in clinical practice. In a meta-analysis of published trials with different classes of antidepressants, including SSRI and tricyclic antidepressants, the small benefit of these drugs on repetitive behavior disappeared after statistical adjustment (Carrasco et al., 2012).

Other types of SSRI were tested in ASD children with stereotypy and repetitive behaviors, for example: fluvoxamine, sertraline, paroxetine, citalopram and escitalopram. There is one unpublished trial of fluvoxamine, which was poorly tolerated by children (McDougle et al., 1996). There are no RCT of sertraline and paroxetine in ASD children (Weinssman & Bridgemohan, 2012). The largest published trial of citalopram (mean dose 16mg/d) found no effect at all on repetitive or compulsive behavior but found a possible effect on challenging behaviors (King et al., 2009). Others RCT didn't show strengths of evidence for effect of citalopram or escitalopram to reduce repetitive or challenging behavior (McPheeters et al., 2011).

Concerning antipsychotic drugs, in the RUPP studies, stereotypies and repetitive behaviors were examined as secondary outcomes and then risperidone achieved levels of statistical significance in reduction of repetitive behavior (McDougle et al., 2005). Similarly, aripiprazole studies showed that the agent significantly improved repetitive behaviors over placebo (Marcus et al., 2009; Owen et al., 2009).

There is only one small RCT which shows the efficacy of valproate in repetitive behaviors of ASD children (Hollander et al., 2006). Our group avoids the usage of valproate in such symptoms. In summary, from the clinical point of view, it is hard to improve stereotypy and repetitive behaviors with pharmacotherapy. As a matter of fact, sometimes these symptoms can be more uncomfortable to parents than patients.

4.4. Mood instability

In clinical practice, mood instability is more difficult to control in ASD patients compared with typically developed children (Gottfried & Riesgo, 2011). Different drugs have been used, including antipsychotics, SSRI, and lithium. The problem is that none of these medications have been studied with RCT specifically for mood regulation in ASD pediatric patients (Weinssman & Bridgemohan, 2012).

If mood lability is associated with disruptive behavior, the best choice could be atypical antipsychotics. If this symptom is associated with depression and or anxiety, the use of SSRI could be considered. It is important to remember the higher possibilities of behavioral activation in ASD patients after SSRI use, leading to hypomaniac states in susceptible children.

4.5. Sleep disorders

Sleep disorders can be identified years before an unequivocal diagnosis of autism. Not infrequently, we face with sleep complaints in very young babies who lately will develop the whole clinical picture compatible with ASD. By the other hand, sleep disorders occur more frequently in ASD patients compared with developing children (Benvenuto et al., 2012; Miano & Ferri, 2010).

Sleep disorders tend to be under-recognized valued in the ASD patient group, probably because they can be considered less disabling than aggression and repetitive behaviors; however, ongoing abnormal sleep patterns are very disruptive to the overall quality of family life and interfere with patient daytime functioning. Parents frequently ask for medication and then physicians are confronted with the lack of FAD-approved treatments for this problem (Kaplan & McCracken, 2012; Weinssman & Bridgemohan, 2012).

Before use of medication, is important to ensure appropriate sleep hygiene as well as to use behavioral intervention. Pharmacology is recommended only when psychosocial treatments fail. Melatonin administration in ASDs is reported to be safe, well tolerated and efficient in improving sleep parameters and daytime behavior, and in decreasing of parental stress (Malow et al., 2011; Rossignol & Frye, 2011).

Core symptoms	Medications	Level of evidence
Aggressiveness	Risperidone*	Large scale double blind RCT
Irritability	Aripiprazole*	Large scale double blind RCT
elf-injury	Olanzapine	Double blind RCT
Other disruptive behaviors	Clozapine	Small open label reports
	Ziprazidone	Small open label reports
	Valproic acid	RCT
	Topiramate	RCT
Hyperactivity	Metilfenidate	Crossover RCT
Inattention	Atomoxetine	Crossover RCT
	Risperidone*	Large scale double blind RCT**
	Aripiprazole*	Large scale double blind RCT**
	Guanfacine	RCT
	Clonidine	Small open label reports
Repetitive behavior	Risperidone*	Large scale double blind RCT**
Stereotypies	Aripiprazole*	Large scale double blind RCT**
	Fluoxetine	RCT
	Valproic acid	RCT
Sleep disorders	Melatonin	RCT

*FDA-approved medications for ASD children; **Secondary analysis; RCT = randomized controlled trials

Table 2. Psychopharmacological treatment in ASD patients

5. Non-medical treatment of ASD patients

The treatment of ASD evolves professionals coming from different area and usually is characterized by comprehensive and intense programs encompassing both patients and families. Early identification is critically important to ensure that families have the opportunity to reap the many unique benefits that may arise from early intervention efforts. For example, intervention efforts that occur early during a child's development may have the advantage of increasing brain plasticity, which may enhance outcomes (LeBlanc & Gillis, 2012).

In our experience, children with low intensity ASD treats, when early-treated can eventually get out from de ASD diagnosis when accessed by CARS, a rating scale of autism symptoms (Gottfried & Riesgo, 2011).

The non-medical intervention programs are directed to the core social, communication and cognitive issues in autism. The objectives of each one program are selected according with the specific abilities and difficulties as well as the actual neurodevelopmental phase of the ASD patient. As a result, this kind of intervention needs to be customized (Dawson & Burner, 2011; LeBlanc & Gillis, 2012).

In general, the following types of therapy can be used both isolate or in different combinations: behavioral, occupational, speech therapy as well as psychopedagogic therapy. Although the non-medical treatments for ASD patients can be different from each other, they usually had the same goals, such as to give the child the best degree of independent functioning as well as to improve quality of life from the patient and family (Myers & Johnson, 2007).

There is a consensus that facing a suspicious case of ASD in children the treatment must be promptly initiated, independently of the type of non-medical treatment, because of the brain plasticity in the developing child (LeBlanc & Gillis, 2012; Lord & McGee, 2001).

Besides the large number of non-medical type of treatment, there are some of them with good level of evidence. According with the National Autism Center's Standard Report, after a systematic review of literature available from 1957 to 2007, at least 11 treatment methods for ASD were considered with good level of evidence.

Additionally, there are some problems in evaluating the efficacy of non-medical treatments in ASD patients. For example, the small sample sizes, the different methodologies, the difficulty in the outcome measures, etc.

5.1. Behavioral treatment

The therapies involving behavioral and educational strategies are the main components of the non-medical treatments of ASD children. The only psychoeducational treatment that meets the criteria as well-established and efficacious intervention for ASD to date is the behavior treatment (Dawson & Burner, 2011; LeBlanc & Gillis, 2012).

There is consensual that behavioral therapy must be intensive with at least 25 hours per week, all year long. There are two main types of behavioral treatments: interventionists and non-interventionists. Among the first group of available therapies, there are three principal methods: a) Applied Behavior Analysis (ABA); b) Treatment and Educational of Autistic and related Communication-handicapped Children (TEACCH); c) developmental/relationship-based therapy (Floortime). Some of these strategies use combinations of different models and are denominated integrative models. To date, there is no evidence that integrative models are better than the original models (Weinssman & Bridgemohan, 2012). By the other side, one example of non-interventionist behavioral therapy is the Picture Exchange Charts System (PECS).

5.1.1. ABA (Applied Behavior Analysis)

Aims to teach the absent child skills through the introduction of these skills in stages. Usually, each one of the skills is individually showed, presenting it coupled with an indication or instruction. When necessary, any support that is offered should be removed as soon as possible. (Ospina et al., 2008; Warren et al., 2011). In the clinical setting, we have identified problems in terms of improvement from the classroom as well as a trend to overestimate the efficacy of ABA.

5.1.2. Treatment and Educational of Autistic and related Communication-handicapped Children (TEACCH)

Use structured activities and environment to help ASD patients to improve compromised area. The model is adapted to each one child and addresses environment organization as well as predicable routines in order to adapt the environment to make it easier for the child to understand it, and understand what is expected of her. TEACCH programs are usually given in a classroom, but can also be made at home. Parents work with professionals as co-therapists for techniques that can be continued at home. It is used by psychologists, special education teachers, speech therapists and trained professionals (Myers & Johnson, 2007).

5.1.3. Floortime

The main objective is to teach fundamental skills expected to the level of development which were not acquired in a given ASD patient age, but to date the efficacy evidences are still inconclusive (Ospina et al., 2008). Our group is conducting an evidence-based research to find out if this treatment is reliable.

5.1.4. Picture Exchange Communication System (PECS)

This non-interventionist behavioral therapy enables non-verbal children to communicate by using figures. PECS can be used at home, in the classroom or in several others environments (Bondy & Frost, 2001). A meta-analysis showed that PECS is a promising intervention (Ganz et al., 2012).

Psychoeducational treatments	Example	Effectiveness
Interventional Models	ABA* TEACCH Denver model Floortime	Well established Insufficient evidence to recommend one over another
Specific behaviors	Focal behavior intervention	Well established
Communication	PECS	Promising results
Social skills instruction		Promising results
Integrative Models	Focal behavior intervention	Insufficient evidence to recommend one over another
Parental role	Parent-mediated intervention programs	Inconsistent results Small size studies
Sensory integration therapy		Inconsistent results
Occupational therapy		Little research

*Suggested by Autism Center Guidelines

Table 3. psychoeducational treatment of ASD patients

5.2. Complementary and alternative therapies

Complementary and alternative medicine (CAM) encompasses different kinds of medical and healthcare systems, practices, and products usually not considered to be a part of the conventional medicine. There are several proposed CAM systems to treat ASD children, but to date still without recognized efficacy by FDA. As a result, they are considered "off label". Interestingly, more than 70% of ASD patients are treated by CAM (Rossignol, 2009).

It is important to note that the definition of CAM is slightly different when used in ASD when compared with other medical disorders. That difference is due the fact of many of the psychoeducational therapies used in ASD children, although not considered conventional medical therapies; they are well accepted methods treating this group of patients.

In terms of scientific support, there are three main groups of CAM: a) promising treatments; b) treatments with some degree of scientific evidence; c) treatments with no scientific proved efficacy to date (Rossignol, 2009).

5.2.1. Promising CAM

These types of treatment showed the highest level of evidence and include music therapy, naltrexone, and acetyl-cholinesterase inhibitors (Rossignol, 2009). Concerning music therapy, there is evidence that it is able to improve social interaction as well as communication skills (Gold et al., 2006; Kim et al., 2008). Our group conducted a RCT using music therapy in ASD patients and we identified the promising effect of this treatment (Gattino et al., 2011). There is a comprehensive RCT been done testing the efficacy of music therapy in ASD patients (Geretsegger et al., 2012).

5.2.2. CAM with little evidence

This group of therapies may include the use of carnitine, ocytocin, vitamin C, tetrahydrobiopterin, adrenergic alfa-2 agonists, hyperbaric oxygen therapy, immune-modulatory treatment, and anti-inflammatory treatment (Rossignol 2009). Caution is needed with the hyperbaric oxygen therapy because of the potential adverse effects, such as barotrauma, reversible myopia, oxygen toxicity, and seizures (Weinssman & Bridgemohan, 2012).

5.2.3. CAM with no proved efficacy to date

Several of the proposed CAM for ASD had no proved efficacy to date, for example: use of carnosine, multi-vitamin and mineral complexes, piracetam, omega-3 fatty acids, selective diets, vitamin B6, magnesium, chelation, cyproheptadine, glutamate antagonists, acupuncture, auditory integration training, massage, neuro-feedback, and others (Rossignol, 2009).

6. Clinical recommendations in ASD

The following clinical recommendations can be done as a result of more than twenty years of personal clinical practice in Child Neurology dealing with ASD children, among other neuropediatric situations. For instance, our Child Neurology Unit (http://www.ufrgs.br/neuropediatria) usually makes more than 16,000 neuropediatric evaluations per year.

From the clinical point of view, it is important to remember the ongoing changes in DSM criteria for ASD diagnosis. To date, we still deal with five different diagnosis of autism, according with DSM-IV criteria. Even after modifications due the new DSM-V classification, ASD children will remain as a heterogeneous group, making difficult the exact clinical diagnosis.

It is important to remember that ASD diagnosis can be catastrophic to parents. As a result, an incorrect diagnosis would be even worse. That is the reason to be careful in terms of making ASD diagnosis as well as to make a double check if diagnosis is really correct.

After finishing a list of the prominent symptoms, the next step is to decide if they are intense enough to deserve treatment, which is not easy. Some symptoms seem to be more unpleasant to parents than the ASD child. At this point, there is no guideline to follow, and the previous clinical experience is extremely helpful.

Usually the non-medical treatment is started earlier than the use of medications. It is important to remember the relevance of evidence-based CAM, since there are a great number of proposed non-medical treatments.

In general, medications are used in addition to non-medical treatments. The best medication approach would be monotherapy, but it is not always possible in the real clinical world. Another critical problem in terms of psychopharmacotherapy is the paucity of well-conducted RCT, as pointed before in this chapter, especially in the table 2. To date, there are only two FDA-approved antipsychotic medications for ASD in children: risperidone and aripiprazole.

Risperidone was approved by FDA in 2006. The usual dose varies from 1 to 3mg/day. In our practice, 3mg/day of risperidone seems to be the cutoff dose in terms of seizure susceptibility. We have identified patients who experienced seizures with doses higher than 3mg/day. Aripiprazole was FDA-approved in 2009 and the daily dose is up to 15mg.

Because of ASD patients are almost twenty times more prone to have epilepsy when compared with normally developing children, and because of many of the drugs used in autism can decrease the seizure threshold in susceptible children, it is important to assure that there is a previous normal EEG before prescribing psychopharmacotherapy.

7. Conclusions and future remarks

The clinical approach includes a general management as well as two types of not excluding treatment strategies: one with medication and another without medication. From the clinical point of view, these two types of treatment are, in fact, complementary.

In the clinical practice, numerous types of treatment have been proposed and there is urgent need to choose any one of them in short period of time. Searching literature, a lack of well conducted RCT was identified. As a result, caution is the best form to approach ASD cases.

Future perspectives in the treatment of ASD probably will include immunomodulation, quantic biochemistry, stem cell therapy and other forms of approach after careful RCT attesting its efficiency.

Author details

Rudimar Riesgo[1,2], Carmem Gottfried[1,3] and Michele Becker[1,2]

1 Translational Research Group in Autism, (UFRGS) Federal University of Rio Grande do Sul, Porto Alegre, RS, Brazil

2 Child Neurology Unit, HCPA (Clinical Hospital of Porto Alegre), UFRGS, Porto Alegre, RS, Brazil

3 Neuroglial Plasticity Laboratory, Department of Biochemistry, Postgraduate Program of Biochemistry, Institute of Basic Health Sciences, UFRGS, Porto Alegre, RS, Brazil

References

[1] Abramson, R. K.,Wright, H.H., Cuccaro, M.L., Lawrence, L.G., Babb, S., Pencarinha, D., Marstelle, F., & Harris, E.C. 1992. Biological liability in families with autism. Journal of the American Academy of Child and Adolescent Psychiatry, 31, 2, pp. 370-1.

[2] Arora, M., Praharaj, S.K., Sarkhel, S., & Sinha, V.K. 2011. Asperger disorder in adults. Southern Medical Journal, 104, 4, pp. 264-8.

[3] Association, American Psychiatric, ed. 2002. Manual Diagnóstico e Estatístico de Transtornos Mentais: DSM-IV-TR. Artmed, Porto Alegre.

[4] Becker, M. M., Wagner, M.B., Bosa, C.A., Schmidt, C., Longo, D., Papaleo, C., & Riesgo, R.S. 2012. Translation and validation of Autism Diagnostic Interview-Revised (ADI-R) for autism diagnosis in Brazil. Arquivos de Neuro-Psiquiatria, 70, 3, pp. 185-90.

[5] Beherec, L., Lambrey, S., Quilici, G., Rosier, A., Falissard, B., & Guillin, O. 2011. Retrospective review of clozapine in the treatment of patients with autism spectrum disorder and severe disruptive behaviors. Journal of Clinical Psychopharmacology, 31, 3, pp. 341-4.

[6] Belsito, K. M., Law, P.A., Kirk, K.S., Landa, R.J., & Zimmerman, A.W. 2001. Lamotrigine therapy for autistic disorder: a randomized, double-blind, placebo-controlled trial. Journal of Autism and Developmental Disorders, 31, 2, pp. 175-81.

[7] Benvenuto, A., Battan, B., Porfirio, M.C., & Curatolo, P. 2012. Pharmacotherapy of autism spectrum disorders. Brain & Development, http://dx.doi.org/10.1016/j.braindev.2012.03.015.

[8] Billstedt, E., Gillberg, I.C., & Gillberg, C. 2005. Autism after adolescence: population-based 13- to 22-year follow-up study of 120 individuals with autism diagnosed in childhood. Journal of Autism and Developmental Disorders, 35, 3, pp. 351-60.

[9] Bondy, A., & Frost, L. 2001. The Picture Exchange Communication System. Behavior Modification, 25, 5, pp. 725-44.

[10] Campbell, M., Anderson, L.T., Small, A.M., Perry, R., Green,W.H., & Caplan, R. 1982. The effects of haloperidol on learning and behavior in autistic children. Journal of Autism and Developmental Disorders, 12, 2, pp. 167-75.

[11] Carrasco, M.,Volkmar, F.R., & Bloch, M.H. 2012. Pharmacologic treatment of repetitive behaviors in autism spectrum disorders: evidence of publication bias. Pediatrics, 129, 5, pp. e1301-10.

[12] Cederlund, M., Hagberg, B., & Gillberg, C. 2010. Asperger syndrome in adolescent and young adult males. Interview, self- and parent assessment of social, emotional, and cognitive problems. Research in Developmental Disabilities, 31, 2, pp. 287-98.

[13] Center, National Autism. 2009. The National Autism Center's National Standards Report [cited 08/23/2012. Available from www.nationalautismcenter.org/pdf/NAC %20Standards%20Report.pdf

[14] Charnsil, C. 2011. Efficacy of atomoxetine in children with severe autistic disorders and symptoms of ADHD: an open-label study. Journal of Attention Disorders, 15, 8, pp. 684-9

[15] Dawson, G., & Burner, K. 2011. Behavioral interventions in children and adolescents with autism spectrum disorder: a review of recent findings. Current Opinion in Pediatrics, 23, 6, pp. 616-20.

[16] Di Martino, A., Melis, G., Cianchetti, C., & Zuddas, A. 2004. Methylphenidate for pervasive developmental disorders: safety and efficacy of acute single dose test and ongoing therapy: an open-pilot study. Journal of Child and Adolescent Psychopharmacology, 14, 2, pp. 207-18.

[17] Gadia, C. A., Tuchman, R., & Rotta, N. T. 2004. Autism and pervasive developmental disorders. Jornal de Pediatria (Rio J), 80, 2, pp. S83-94.

[18] Gadow, K. D., DeVincent, C. J., & Pomeroy, J. 2006. ADHD symptom subtypes in children with pervasive developmental disorder. Journal of Autism and Developmental Disorders, 36, 2, pp. 271-83.

[19] Ganz, J. B., Davis, J.L., Lund, E.M., Goodwyn, F.D., & Simpson, R.L. 2012. Meta-analysis of PECS with individuals with ASD: investigation of targeted versus non-targeted outcomes, participant characteristics, and implementation phase. Research in Developmental Disabilities, 33, 2, pp. 406-18.

[20] Gattino, G., Riesgo, R., Longo, D., Leite, J.L., & Faccini, L.S. 2011. Effect of relational music therapy of communication of children with autism: a randomized controlled study. Nordic Journal of Music Therapy, 20, 2, pp.142-154.

[21] Geretsegger, M., Holck, U., & Gold, C. 2012. Randomised controlled trial of improvisational music therapy's effectiveness for children with autism spectrum disorders (TIME-A): study protocol. BMC Pediatrics, 5, 12, pp. 2.

[22] Gold, C., Wigram, T., & Elefant, C. 2006. Music therapy for autistic spectrum disorder. Cochrane database of systematic reviews, 2, CD004381.

[23] Gottfried, C., & Riesgo, R. 2011. Antipsychotics in the treatment of autism. In Autism spectrum disorders: from genes to environment, T. Williams, Intech: Rijeka. pp.23-46

[24] Handen, B.L., Sahl, R., & Hardan, A.Y. 2008. Guanfacine in children with autism and/or intellectual disabilities. Journal of Developmental and Behavioral Pediatrics, 29, 4, pp. 303-8.

[25] Hardan, A.Y., Jou, R.J., & Handen, B.L. 2004. A retrospective assessment of topiramate in children and adolescents with pervasive developmental disorders. Journal of Child and Adolescent Psychopharmacology, 14, 3, pp. 426-32.

[26] Hofvander, B., Delorme, R., Chaste, P., Nyden, A., Wentz, E., Stahlberg, O., Herbrecht, E., Stopin, A., Anckarsater, H., Gillberg, C., Rastam, M., & Leboyer, M. 2009. Psychiatric and psychosocial problems in adults with normal-intelligence autism spectrum disorders. BMC Psychiatry, 9, pp. 35.

[27] Hollander, E., Chaplin, W., Soorya, L., Wasserman, S., Novotny, S., Rusoff, J., Feirsen, N., Pepa, L., & Anagnostou, E. 2010. Divalproex sodium vs placebo for the treatment of irritability in children and adolescents with autism spectrum disorders. Neuropsychopharmacology : official publication of the American College of Neuropsychopharmacology, 35, 4, pp. 990-8.

[28] Hollander, E., Soorya, L.,Wasserman, S., Esposito, K., Chaplin, W., & Anagnostou, E. 2006. Divalproex sodium vs. placebo in the treatment of repetitive behaviours in autism spectrum disorder. The international journal of neuropsychopharmacology / official scientific journal of the Collegium Internationale Neuropsychopharmacologicum, 9, 2, pp. 209-13.

[29] Howlin, P., Goode, S., Hutton, J., & Rutter, M. 2004. Adult outcome for children with autism. Journal of child psychology and psychiatry, and allied disciplines, 45, 2, pp. 212-29.

[30] Howlin, P., Mawhood, L., & Rutter, M. 2000. Autism and developmental receptive language disorder--a follow-up comparison in early adult life. II: Social, behavioural, and psychiatric outcomes. Journal of child psychology and psychiatry, and allied disciplines, 41,5, pp. 561-78.

[31] Jahromi, L.B., Kasari, C.L., McCracken, J.T., Lee, L.S., Aman, M.G., McDougle, C.J., Scahill, L., Tierney, E., Arnold, L.E., Vitiello, B., Ritz, L., Witwer, A., Kustan, E., Ghuman, J., & Posey, D.J. 2009. Positive effects of methylphenidate on social communication and self-regulation in children with pervasive developmental disorders and hyperactivity. Journal of Autism and Developmental Disorders, 39, 3, pp. 395-404.

[32] Jaselskis, C.A., Cook, E.H., Fletcher, Jr., K.E., & Leventhal, B.L.1992. Clonidine treatment of hyperactive and impulsive children with autistic disorder. Journal of Clinical Psychopharmacology, 12, 5, pp. 322-7.

[33] Kanne, S.M., & Mazurek, M.O. 2011. Aggression in children and adolescents with ASD: prevalence and risk factors. Journal of Autism and Developmental Disorders, 41, 7, pp. 926-37.

[34] Kanner, L. 1943. Autistic disturbances of affective contact. Nervous Child, 2, pp. 217-250.

[35] Kaplan, G., & McCracken, J.T. 2012. Psychopharmacology of autism spectrum disorders. Pediatric Clinics of North America, 59, 1, pp. 175-87.

[36] Kim, J., Wigram, T., & Gold, C. 2008. The effects of improvisational music therapy on joint attention behaviors in autistic children: a randomized controlled study. Journal of Autism and Developmental Disorders, 38, 9, pp. 1758-66.

[37] Kim, Y.S., Leventhal, B.L., Koh,Y.J., Fombonne, E., Laska, E., Lim, E.C., Cheon, K.A., Kim, S.J., Kim, Y.K., Lee, H., Song, D.H., & Grinker, R.R. 2011. Prevalence of autism spectrum disorders in a total population sample. The American Journal of Psychiatry, 168, 9, pp. 904-12.

[38] King, B.H., Hollander, E., Sikich, L., McCracken, J.T., Scahill, L., Bregman, J.D., Donnelly, C.L., Anagnostou, E., Dukes, K., Sullivan, L., Hirtz, D.,Wagner, A., & Ritz, L. 2009. Lack of efficacy of citalopram in children with autism spectrum disorders and high levels of repetitive behavior: citalopram ineffective in children with autism. Archives of General Psychiatry, 66, 6, pp. 583-90.

[39] LeBlanc, L.A., & Gillis, J.M. 2012. Behavioral interventions for children with autism spectrum disorders. Pediatric Clinics of North America, 59, 1, pp. 147-64.

[40] Leekam, S.R., Prior, M.R., & Uljarevic, M. 2011. Restricted and repetitive behaviors in autism spectrum disorders: a review of research in the last decade. Psychological Bulletin, 137, 4, pp. 562-93.

[41] Longo, D., Schuler-Faccini, L., Brandalize, A.P., Riesgo, R.S., & Bau, C.H. 2009. Influence of the 5-HTTLPR polymorphism and environmental risk factors in a Brazilian sample of patients with autism spectrum disorders. Brain Res, 1267, pp. 9-17.

[42] Lord, C., & McGee, J.P. eds. 2001. Educating children with autism. Washington, DC: National Academy Press.

[43] Malone, R.P., Delaney, M.A., Hyman, S.B., & Cater, J.R. 2007. Ziprasidone in adolescents with autism: an open-label pilot study. Journal of Child and Adolescent Psychopharmacolog, 17, 6, pp. 779-90.

[44] Malow, B., Adkins, K.W., McGrew, S.G., Wang, L., Goldman, S.E., Fawkes, D., & Burnette, C. 2011. Melatonin for sleep in children with autism: a controlled trial examining dose, tolerability, and outcomes. Journal of Autism and Developmental Disorders, 42, 8, pp. 1729-37.

[45] Marcus, R.N., Owen, R., Kamen, L., Manos, G., McQuade, R.D., Carson, W.H., & Aman, M.G. 2009. A placebo-controlled, fixed-dose study of aripiprazole in children and adolescents with irritability associated with autistic disorder. Journal of the American Academy of Child and Adolescent Psychiatry, 48, 11, pp. 1110-9.

[46] Mawhood, L., Howlin, P., & Rutter, M. 2000. Autism and developmental receptive language disorder--a comparative follow-up in early adult life. I: Cognitive and language outcomes. Journal of child psychology and psychiatry, and allied disciplines, 41, 5, pp. 547-59.

[47] Mazzone, L., & Ruta, L. 2006. Topiramate in children with autistic spectrum disorders. Brain & Development, 28, 10, pp. 668.

[48] McCracken, J.T., McGough, J., Shah, B., Cronin, P., Hong, D., Aman, M.G., Arnold, L.E., Lindsay, R., Nash, P., Hollway, J., McDougle, C.J., Posey, D., Swiezy, N., Kohn, A.,

Scahill, L., Martin, A., Koenig, K., Volkmar, F., Carroll, D., Lancor, A., Tierney, E., Ghuman, J., Gonzalez, N.M., Grados, M.,Vitiello, B., Ritz, L., Davies, M., Robinson, J., & McMahon, D. 2002. Risperidone in children with autism and serious behavioral problems. The New England Journal of Medicine, 347, 5, pp. 314-21.

[49] McDougle, C.J., Naylor, S.T., Cohen, D.J., Volkmar, F.R., Heninger, G.R., & Price, L.H. 1996. A double-blind, placebo-controlled study of fluvoxamine in adults with autistic disorder. Archives of General Psychiatry, 53, 11, pp. 1001-8.

[50] McDougle, C.J., Scahill, L., Aman, M.G., McCracken, J.T., Tierney, E., Davies, M., Arnold, L.E., Posey, D.J., Martin, A., Ghuman, J.K., Shah, B., Chuang, S.Z., Swiezy, N.B., Gonzalez, N.M., Hollway, J., Koenig, K., McGough, J.J., Ritz, L., &Vitiello, B. 2005. Risperidone for the core symptom domains of autism: results from the study by the autism network of the research units on pediatric psychopharmacology. The American Journal of Psychiatry,62, 6, pp. 1142-8.

[51] McPheeters, M.L., Warren, Z., Sathe, N., Bruzek, J.L., Krishnaswami, S., Jerome, R.N., & Veenstra-Vanderweele,V. 2011. A systematic review of medical treatments for children with autism spectrum disorders. Pediatrics, 127, 5, pp. e1312-21.

[52] Miano, S., & Ferri, R. 2010. Epidemiology and management of insomnia in children with autistic spectrum disorders. Paediatric Drugs, 12, 2, pp. 75-84.

[53] Ming, X., Gordon, E., Kang, N., & Wagner, G.C. 2008. Use of clonidine in children with autism spectrum disorders. Brain & Development, 30, 7, pp. 454-60.

[54] Miral, S., Gencer, O., Inal-Emiroglu, F.N., Baykara, B., Baykara, A., & Dirik, E. 2008. Risperidone versus haloperidol in children and adolescents with AD : a randomized, controlled, double-blind trial. European Child & Adolescent Psychiatry, 17, 1, pp. 1-8.

[55] Murray, M.J. 2010. Attention-deficit/Hyperactivity Disorder in the context of Autism spectrum disorders. Current Psychiatry Reports, 12, 5, pp. 382-8.

[56] Myers, S. M., & Johnson, C.P. 2007. Management of children with autism spectrum disorders. Pediatrics, 120, 5, pp. 1162-82.

[57] Nikolov, R., Jonker, J., & Scahill, L. 2006. Autistic disorder: current psychopharmacological treatments and areas of interest for future developments. Revista Brasileira de Psiquiatria, 28, Suppl 1, pp. S39-46.

[58] Ospina, M.B., Krebs Seida, J., Clark, B., Karkhaneh, M., Hartling, L., Tjosvold, L., Vandermeer, B., & Smith, V. 2008. Behavioural and developmental interventions for autism spectrum disorder: a clinical systematic review. PloS one, 3,11, pp. e3755.

[59] Owen, R., Sikich, L., Marcus, R.N., Corey-Lisle, P., Manos, G., McQuade, R.D., Carson,W.H., & Findling, R.L. 2009. Aripiprazole in the treatment of irritability in children and adolescents with autistic disorder. Pediatrics, 124, 6, pp. 1533-40.

[60] Pereira, A., Riesgo, R.S., & Wagner, M.B. 2008. Childhood autism: translation and validation of the Childhood Autism Rating Scale for use in Brazil. Jornal de Pediatria (Rio J), 84, 6, pp. 487-94.

[61] Piven, J., Harper, J., Palmer, P., & Arndt, S. 1996. Course of behavioral change in autism: a retrospective study of high-IQ adolescents and adults. Journal of the American Academy of Child and Adolescent Psychiatry, 35, 4, pp. 523-9.

[62] Posey, D.J., Aman, M.G., McCracken, J.T., Scahill, L., Tierney, E., Arnold, L.E., Vitiello, B., Chuang, S.Z., Davies, M., Ramadan,Y., Witwer, A.N., Swiezy, N.B., Cronin, P., Shah, B., Carroll, D.H., Young, C., Wheeler, C., & McDougle, C.J. 2007. Positive effects of methylphenidate on inattention and hyperactivity in pervasive developmental disorders: an analysis of secondary measures. Biological Psychiatry, 61, 4, pp. 538-44.

[63] Potenza, M.N., Holmes, J.P., Kanes, S.J., & McDougle, C.J. 1999. Olanzapine treatment of children, adolescents, and adults with pervasive developmental disorders: an open-label pilot study. Journal of Clinical Psychopharmacology, 19,1, pp. 37-44.

[64] Quincozes-Santos, A., Bobermin, L.D., Tonial, R.P., Bambini-Junior, V., Riesgo, R., & Gottfried, C. 2010. Effects of atypical (risperidone) and typical (haloperidol) antipsychotic agents on astroglial functions. European Archives of Psychiatry and Clinical Neuroscience, 260, 6, pp. 475-81.

[65] Rezaei, V., Mohammadi, M.R., Ghanizadeh, A., Sahraian, A., Tabrizi, M., Rezazadeh, S.A., & Akhondzadeh, S. 2010. Double-blind, placebo-controlled trial of risperidone plus topiramate in children with autistic disorder. Progress in Neuro-Psychopharmacology & Biological Psychiatry, 34, 7, pp. 1269-72.

[66] Rommelse, N.N., Franke, B.,Geurts, H.M., Hartman, C.A., & Buitelaar, J.K. 2010. Shared heritability of attention-deficit/hyperactivity disorder and autism spectrum disorder. European Child & Adolescent Psychiatry, 19, 3, pp. 281-95.

[67] Rossignol, D.A. 2009. Novel and emerging treatments for autism spectrum disorders: a systematic review. Annals of Clinical Psychiatry : official journal of the American Academy of Clinical Psychiatrists, 21,4, pp. 213-36.

[68] Rossignol, D.A., & Frye, R.E. 2011. Melatonin in autism spectrum disorders: a systematic review and meta-analysis. Developmental Medicine and Child Neurology, 53, 9, pp. 783-92.

[69] RUPP. 2005. Randomized, controlled, crossover trial of methylphenidate in pervasive developmental disorders with hyperactivity. Archives of General Psychiatry, 62, 11, pp. 1266-74.

[70] Rutter, M., Greenfeld, D., & Lockyer, L. 1967. A five to fifteen year follow-up study of infantile psychosis. II. Social and behavioural outcome. The British Journal of Psychiatry : the journal of mental science, 113, 504, pp. 1183-99.

[71] Scahill, L., Aman, M.G., McDougle, C.J., McCracken, J.T., Tierney, E., Dziura, J., Arnold, L.E., Posey, D., Young, C., Shah, B., Ghuman, J., Ritz, L., & Vitiello, B. 2006. A prospec-

tive open trial of guanfacine in children with pervasive developmental disorders. Journal of Child and Adolescent Psychopharmacology, 16, 5, pp. 589-98.

[72] Seltzer, M.M., Krauss, M.W., Shattuck, P.T., Orsmond, G., Swe, A., & Lord, C. 2003. The symptoms of autism spectrum disorders in adolescence and adulthood. Journal of Autism and Developmental Disorders, 33, 6, pp. 565-81.

[73] Stahlberg, O., Soderstrom, H., Rastam, M., & Gillberg, C. 2004. Bipolar disorder, schizophrenia, and other psychotic disorders in adults with childhood onset AD/HD and/or autism spectrum disorders. Journal of Neural Transmission, 111, 7, pp. 891-902.

[74] Szatmari, P., Archer, L., Fisman, S., Streiner, D.L., and Wilson, F. 1995. Asperger's syndrome and autism: differences in behavior, cognition, and adaptive functioning. Journal of the American Academy of Child and Adolescent Psychiatry, 34, 12, pp. 1662-71.

[75] Warren, Z., McPheeters, M. L., Sathe, N., Foss-Feig, J.H., Glasser, A., & Veenstra-Vanderweele, J. 2011. A systematic review of early intensive intervention for autism spectrum disorders. Pediatrics, 127, 5, pp. e1303-11.

[76] Weinssman, L., & Bridgemohan, C. 2012. (last updated: 06/05/2012) Autism spectrum disorder in children and adolescents: pharmacologic interventions. In, *Up To Date*, acessed on 08/30/2012, Available from http://www.uptodate.com/contents-autism-spectrum-disorders-in -children-and-adolescents-pharmacological-interventions

[77] Zeiner, P., Gjevik, E., and Weidle, B. 2011. Response to atomoxetine in boys with high-functioning autism spectrum disorders and attention deficit/hyperactivity disorder. Acta Paediatrica, 100, 9, pp. 1258-61.

Chapter 4

Addressing Communication Difficulties of Parents of Children of the Autism Spectrum

Fernanda Dreux Miranda Fernandes,
Cibelle Albuquerque de La Higuera Amato,
Danielle Azarias Defense-Netvral,
Juliana Izidro Balestro and
Daniela Regina Molini-Avejonas

Additional information is available at the end of the chapter

1. Introduction

The autism spectrum includes major developmental disorders that, by definition, involve early and severe disorders in the areas of social, communicative and cognitive development. The resulting disorders are frequently severe and persistent with large individual variations. Therefore its impact on the families should not be overlooked.

On the other hand, the intervention aimed towards children with Autism Spectrum Disorders (ASD) should be comprehensive, intensive and long term. It leads to the notion that the families' participation in these processes should be a systematic focus of therapeutic proposals and studies involving children of the autism spectrum.

However, a recent literature review [1] about the papers published in three of the most important journals with specific focus on autism revealed a different reality. Only 0.7% of the papers published between 2005 and 2009 referred to studies about families with ASD children, comprising a total of 4883 participants. It is interesting to note that more than half of the papers about families with children of the autism spectrum were published in the last 18 months of the considered period. The themes of those studies involved issues about stress and emotional problems (13 papers); support groups and quality of life (7 papers); characterization of the families and their members (7 papers); intervention processes and their results (5 papers) and how the parents consider their children with autism spectrum disorders (8 papers).

The growing interest in the area may be a result of the recognition that families should be included in any plan for intervention designed towards ASD children. A recently published research [2] studied the experiences that were shared by families during the diagnostic process that identified an ASD. Reports about 16 children identified that there was an average 2-year lag between the first doubts about the child's development and the ASD diagnosis. These processes were more difficult and more painful to families of older children.

Another recent study [3] assessed schooling problems of ASD children and their families. The results confirmed the difficulties frequently observed in adaptation of ASD children in regular schools. The authors point out that opportunities for establishing friendship groups and peer acceptance seem to be the key elements to successful adaptations. [4] studied the opinion of parents of ASD children in the search for treatments - a process that often demands time, money and energy - in six different countries. The most significant issues that emerged were the effectiveness of treatments, relationships with professionals, access to treatments, costs, medication and stress. Early inclusion in a regular school, whenever possible, should be part of the resources provided for the development of children with autism spectrum disorders.

A Brazilian study [5] proposed a questionnaire to the identification of perceptions of caregivers of ASD children about the quality of their communication with their children, regardless of the concrete disorders presented by the child and the specific diagnosis within the spectrum. The questionnaire had a specific focus on the caregivers and was divided in four domains regarding their impressions about themselves, about other people, about their children and about their attitudes with their children. Caregivers report difficulties with other people's reactions to their children's behavior, communicative stile of the adult-child dyad, concern about the child's future and the need for more information about their child communication and instructions on how to face their difficulties.

The atypical communication development of individuals with ASD is related to difficulties with the various communicative roles (as speaker and as listener); disorders in the use of the different communicative means; a restricted repertoire of communicative functions; lack or few demonstrations of communicative intent, imitation, joint attention and other disorders in the social cognitive and symbolic development and social communicative adaptation [6, 7].

Verbal communication may be absent. Language delays, discursive or narrative disorders may also be observed. Social impairments may also vary from lack of visual contact or social reciprocity to severe behavior disorders (including aggressive and disruptive behaviors and eating and sleeping idiosyncrasies).

The aim of this chapter is to present some specific points and strategies to cope with autistic children's communication inabilities and suggestions on how to improve opportunities for communicative development and improvement. Not all the suggestions will be useful to all parents at any moment of their child's development; but probably some of them will answer to doubts of many parents at some point. Hopefully they will help parents and caregivers of ASD children to think about how their child communicates, which can be the key elements of successful communication experiences and the triggers of critical situations. This way they will be able to increase the occurrence of good and pleasant communication while decreasing the number of stressful situations. However, it should be remembered that some amount of misunderstanding and frustrating communicative situations is part of the everyday life of every person and therefore it is not reasonable to plan to completely eliminate them form the ASD child's communicative experiences.

2. Specific focus and action options

The broad themes considered address possible strategies to improve opportunities for communication, favor language development, improve social contact and improve the quality of communication with family and peers.

2.1. Improve opportunities for communication

Observing the communicative style of the ASD child parents may identify new ways of fostering the development of new abilities and their use in different situations or with different functions.

Identifying if there are specific situations when the child uses preferentially a certain communicative mean (speech, gestures, vocalizations, writing).

Showing the possibilities of expressing a certain meaning - or improving the communication's efficiency - by the use of alternative communicative means or by the combination of more than one mean.

Stimulating the use of new gestures, sounds or words in familiar situations.

Depending on the child's abilities, it may be important to exercise various situations and opportunities for expressing a certain content or intent.

In other situations it may be important to improve the creativity in communication. Sometimes it can be useful to show, in familiar situations, the various forms to express a certain message or intent.

Visual contact requires a delicate balance where the person must look at other people but shouldn't stare at them. Parents should be supportive in the development of strategies to improve social visual contact. Simple strategies, as being at the child's eye level, consistently maintaining and requesting eye contact and responding to the child's eye contact initiatives may produce significant results to the child's social adaptation.

Being aware of all the communication the child expresses, regardless of the communicative mean. Shouts, murmurs, vocalizations and gestures may convey meaningful contents and therefore lead to productive interactions. On the other hand, if a communicative attempt made by the child is ignored it may send a confusing feedback about communication strategies and their results.

Exploring natural and routine situations (such as baths, meals, outings) to increase the repertoire of words and expressions that constitute the common ground for communication.

2.2. Stimulate language development

Simple but consistent activities and attitudes may have an important role in building an environment that will stimulate language development and provide comfortable contexts where the child may use his/her communication abilities.

Defining a time or a place to be with the child in a pleasant situation (playing, talking, exchanging impressions about something that happened during the day or planning a future event or activity). The situations should be simple enough so they can happen every day. Its duration may depend on the participants' interest, but should not vary too much, so the child may be comfortable, knowing what will happen next. If the mother has more time during daily routines, she can spend, for example, two fifteen-minute periods playing, talking or working on a project with the child. But if she is overwhelmed by the routine, the father may include these activities in his routine. If both parents are available, the three may be involved in the activities. Siblings and other relatives (even pets) may be included. What is essential is to consider that these short periods of time should be part of a routine that the whole family respects and enjoys.

Adapting adult's language to the child's level of understanding. Sometimes the ASD child present a speech level far superior to his/her understanding level. Parents should consider how well the child understands language and adapt their own language to it.

Associating language to actions (movements of body or objects) or sensorial experiences, such as sounds, smells or tactile sensations (especially those associated with extremes and graduations between them; for example, hot, warm, cold and freezing) will improve the whole experience and therefore increase its meaning.

Waiting for the child's own time to answer a question or perform a task. Also being aware to the fact that sometimes the child will perform a requested action or answer to a question after a quite large time-gap. It can be useful to retrieve the question or the request and show the child if it is still meaningful of if it lost its function. *For example: the mother is cooking, asks the child to get a spoon but when the child doesn't do it immediately she goes and get it - and it is reasonable that it should occur on a natural situation - ; if the child gets the spoon some minutes later the mother should appraise it, thank for the help, but also tell the child that she needed it a few minutes before, or the food would get burned.*

Using linguistic expressions in natural situations while enjoying an activity, such as *one, two, three, go!*; or *bye, bye*; or pick-a-boo. Using onomatopoeic sounds when playing with animals, vehicles or other objects with characteristic sounds, or when telling stories.

Use routine situations such as baths, meals or organizing a drawer to use known and new words and expressions, building a repertoire of words or expressions that will be always used during these situations. For example, always saying *wash both feet* during the bath; *ate it all* when finishing a meal; *socks go together* when organizing a drawer. But also sometimes introducing new elements to familiar situations, for example saying *use your hands to wash both feet*, or *I ate it all, my bely is full* or *socks go together and boxers (or panties) on the other side.*

Use varied and even exaggerated facial expressions, associating them with communicative functions, demonstrating awareness to the child's facial expressions, commenting about them, identifying different facial expressions in pictures and films.

Stimulate the child to use language to express his/her own emotions.

2.3. Improve social contact

When the family engages in social activities and includes the ASD child in them, there are more opportunities for social interaction. Sharing social situations with their ASD child parents will be able to eventually identify focus of more difficulties and also productive strategies to help the child to cope with them.

Taking the child to parks and playgrounds and stimulating the child to interact with other children. Situations such as sharing a swing, respecting the line for the slide or playing on the sand along with other children, may provide interesting and pleasant experiences that can represent opportunities to experience communicative strategies and exercise recently acquired abilities. Parents should be aware however, that cooperative and competitive activities are frequently stressful and cause of major disagreement between children with normal development also. Said disagreements are also important experiences to the development of social and communicative repertoires as long as they are accompanied by a soothing and supportive attitude by the parents.

Including the child in family activities such as travels, outings, visits to different places and social activities. Planning these activities with the child will help him/her to prepare for new situations, talking about what to expect, how to react in specific contexts. Including relaxing time and places to unwind or calm down will probably be useful to the whole family and can be adjusted to each child's needs and rhythm.

Helping the child to cope with problematic places and situations. Do not avoiding stressful situations but trying to identify and reduce the stressing factors. They may be related to loud noises, flashing light, crowds, specific characters (such as clowns or Santa Claus) or previous unpleasant experiences. Parents should try gradual approximation to the situations, explaining the source of lights and sounds, increasing time or proximity according to the child's response.

Including the child in household routine activities. The child should share house chores as all other family members. Depending to his/her abilities and on the family's routine, the child may unpack shopping bags, organize a drawer, write the shopping list, sort out mailing, measure the dog's food or taking it for a walk. This routine should be part of the child's responsibilities as well as an opportunity to a feeling of accomplishment.

2.4. Improve the quality of interaction within the family and with peers

Attention to the child's interests, interactive strategies, communication breaks or triggers to disruptive behavior may enable parents to improve the quality of the family's interaction. All must be willing to proceed to changes in routines, responses and automatic reactions.

Observing and identifying child's interests, behaviour and communicative attempts are essential to attribute effective value to the interaction and to respond to it in a productive way, building contexts of joint attention and shared experiences.

Including the child in the family's dynamic means to comply with the same rules and limits that are applied to the other members. But close observation may also indicate that for some children more clear routines and limits may be useful. An agreement about a sequence of activities (such as choosing a toy or game, playing with it and storing it away when finished) may help the child to organize his/her expectations. Specific strategies may be needed to maintain the agreed procedure, but it may be essential to be consistent with it until the child can build his/her own rhythm and behavioural organization.

In the presence of peers (siblings, cousins, friends' children) take advantage of the opportunity to encourage the child to share objects and toys and to respect collective rules (waiting for his/her turn, complying with rules of specific games or sports).

Use unexpected situations to help the child to learn how to cope with them. Depending on the child's level, it can involve: searching for a lost item, fixing a broken toy, asking for help when needed or arguing a point of view.

Encourage the child to engage in organized activities or combinatory play, such as building blocks, puzzles, logical sequences of pictures, narrating stories. Using concepts as time, space, rhythm and position.

Use and encourage the combined use of speech and gestures and facial expressions to improve communicative efficiency.

Try to adapt the length and complexity of phrases and language to the child's language level and to guarantee the child's attention (using eye contact, physical contact of other sensory clue to the communicative situation).

Be aware of the result of your communicative initiatives, as shown by the child's reactions or answers. Try to identify what are the most difficult points to the child's comprehension and be prepared to communicative breaks and alternatives to solve them.

3. Conclusions

The suggestions presented are mostly examples on how everyday life activities and routines can be used to increase the opportunities to improve the ASD child's communicative abilities and their creative use as an important part of the whole development.

The notion that the family's routine is an important part of the child's developmental environment, however, should not lead parents or other family members to transform it on a permanent training field. The best intentions and the undeniable stress involved in wishing to provide the better developmental opportunities to their ASD child may result on a stressful and over-stimulating situation. It will probably increase the stress level of the whole family decreasing the opportunities for relaxed, joyful interaction with affectively meaningful persons, which is also very important to the child's development.

The inclusion of parents and other family members in the education and intervention processes with ASD children should not be a responsibility attributed just to therapists or educators. Families can have an active part in it, by asking questions and demanding for instructions.

However, families can also need a "time-out" when they are not requested to collaborate on any structured activity. Each family should be allowed and encouraged to develop its own coping strategies and supported when a more direct approach is needed.

Groups of parents of children attending the same service or going to the same school can be very helpful in building a supportive network that includes persons that share similar problems and may also share some solutions.

Author details

Fernanda Dreux Miranda Fernandes*, Cibelle Albuquerque de La Higuera Amato,
Danielle Azarias Defense-Netvral, Juliana Izidro Balestro and
Daniela Regina Molini-Avejonas

*Address all correspondence to: fernandadreux@usp.br

Department of Phisical Therapy, Speech-Language Pathology and Audiology and Ocupational Therapy, School of Medicine, Universidade de São Paulo, São Paulo, Brazil

References

[1] Fernandes FD. Families with autistic children: international literature. Rev Soc Bras Fonoaudiol. 2009; 14(3): 427-32.

[2] Sansosti FK, Lavik KB, Sansosti JM. Family Experiences through the Autism Diagnostic Process. Focus on Autism and Other Developmental Disabilities, 2012. 27 (2): 81-92 doi 10.1177/1088357612446860

[3] Dillon GV, Underwood JDM. Parental Perspectives of Students with Autism Spectrum Disorders Transitioning from Primary to Secondary School in the United King-

dom. Focus on Autism and Other Developmental Disabilities, 2012. 27(2): 111-121. doi 10.1177/1088357612441827

[4] Mackintosh VH, Goin-Kochel RP, Myers BJ. What do you Like/Dislike about the Treatments you're Currently Using? A Qualitative Study of Parents of Children with Autism Spectrum Disorders. Focus on Autism and Other Developmental Disabilities, 2012. 27: 51-60. doi 1

[5] Balestro JI, Fernandes FDM. Questionnaire about communicative difficulties perceived by parents of ASD children. Rev Soc Bras Fonoaudiol. 2012; 14:

[6] Fernanda FDM, Amato CAH, Molini-Avejonas DR. Language Assessment in Autism in Mohammad-Reza M (ed) A comprehensive Book on autism Spectrum Disorders. Ryjeka: Intech; 2011. p1-20.

[7] Hurlbutt KS. Experiences of Parents who Homeschool their Children with Autism Spectrum Disorders. Focus on Autism and Other Developmental Disabilities. 2011; 26(4): 239- 249, doi 101177/1088357611421170

Chapter 5

Building an Alternative Communication System for Literacy of Children with Autism (SCALA) with Context-Centered Design of Usage

Liliana Maria Passerino and Maria Rosangela Bez

Additional information is available at the end of the chapter

1. Introduction

Human language is a system of linguistic symbols acquired through a long ontological process of cultural learning [1]. It serves two functional aspects, communication and cognition [2]. The communicative function of language emerges in the indicative function and allows the establishment of the communication process through choice and combination of symbols [2], whereas, the cognitive function of language allows the representation of beliefs and intentions through linguistic symbols; thus, acts on one's own mental states and that of others [1]. Our view of autism and the way it affect communication is discussed along those lines.

As our conception of language development, it is assumed that communicating is more than speaking. Communicating means skillfully using a powerful tool of mediation[1]:human language. In addition, human language is taken here with all its possible modes of expression, including verbal and non-verbal symbols. Communication is neither regarded as a linear process of direct use of a symbolic system (language) nor as a process of language acquisition of grammatical and phonetic items. The complex process behind language acquisition includes social, cultural, historical, and intersubjective dimensions and is interactional in essence. Interaction, the fuel for development, occurs within scenes of joint attention, in which interacting agents intentionally use linguistic symbols to express intentions, beliefs and representations from their own perspective in several ways [3]. These are the premises underlying our research.

1 From a sociohistorical perspective, mediation is regarded as a scene of joint attention [1] between two or more subjects intentionally using tools and signs (such as language) to promote a process of appropriation with differentiated responsibility and competence among participants.

Human primates' natural trend to understand others as intentional agents with goals and perceptions is the basis for the engagement in collaborative activities and joint attention [1]. Different from other primates, humans have developed a specific capacity to share attention and establish a unique type of social interaction. Hence, scenes of joint attention constitute social interactional processes in which: 1) agents are reciprocally responsible; 2) there is a shared goal, that is, each partner is aware of the goal to be achieved together; and, 3) participants coordinate their plans of action and intentions mutually so that each participant can anticipate the roles in the interaction and potentially help others with their role if necessary[2] [4].

Scenes of joint attention contribute with the *locus* for the negotiation needed for the construction of intersubjective and perspectivated meanings [1]. This is what characterizes the process of communication as a relational and systemic phenomenon. Subjects are actively involved in interaction with a particular dynamics of implicit or explicit rules over which none of the subjects have complete control.

Such intersubjective and perspectivated construction of meanings reveals the uniqueness of human language as, upon the specific use of a particular linguistic symbol, it carries a local, historical and social meaning jointly constructed. This is also to say that in each interaction, participants quickly update possible meanings.

By extension, learning a language is a process situated relationally, historically and culturally. In each interactional process where two individuals engage, there is an intersubjective reconstruction of the perspectives of the others in the representation of their own intentions and beliefs, which requires interacting individuals to select, filter and reconfigure symbols, according to the context, intentions, beliefs and mental representations of co-participants in the communication process.

Communication implies reorganization and coordination of social, cultural and mental representations of subjects in interaction. It is precisely by means of linguistic symbols, namely signs, that it is possible to build and share meanings. That dialectical dimension of the use/understanding/acquisition of a sign is a feature of the linguistic symbol which always involves two dimensions, language and thought. As a consequence, the attainment of a linguistic symbol constitutes a real and complex act of thought, represented by the word. It is not simply acquired by memorization or association [2].

Language acquisition is realized through the use of the symbol in actions of mediation (triadic) by which participants negotiate and construct meaning in an intersubjective way, because "[...] the meaning of a word is given through the process of verbal and social interaction with adults. Children do not build their own concepts freely. They derive them through the process of understanding the speech of others " [5] (p. 121). It is precisely within those triadic scenes, called joint attention scenes [1], that the interlocutors share some Aspect of their context[3] and where intersubjectivity occurs [4]. It is also important to note that interlocutors may reach different levels intersubjectivity depending on the extent of their exchanges [5, 6].

2 Especially in interactions between subjects with different levels of experience or knowledge about the situation.

3 The context refers to the way objects and events are represented and meant in a situation [6].

Besides intersubjectivity, linguistic symbols require an ability to understand perspectivation. Understanding a symbol is a prerequisite to understanding the intentions, beliefs and background knowledge of others, as well as a particular perspective about an object or event that is incorporated into the symbol [1]. Human ability to adopt different perspectives for the same symbol or to treat different objects as if they were the same for some communicative purpose is only possible because all of those perspectives are incorporated into the symbol. So, this perspectivated nature of linguistic symbols sets forth an endless array of possibilities to manipulate the attention of others with implications for the nature of its cognitive representation [1].

2. Communication in autism: Some considerations

Autism belongs in the group of Pervasive Developmental Disorders (PDDs). Literature highlights a triad of elements [7] for the identification of the disorder: behavior, social interaction, and language and communication [8]. In the presence of autism, such elements portray qualitative features which prove to be peculiar or bear deficits. This session aims at discussing the characteristics related to communication and language in autism in more detail without deepening other inter-related aspects of the syndrome (such as interaction and behavior). Presenting a state of the art of on autism is not intended here, but rather, a brief review of some researches concerning language use and communication.

The field of language and communication in autism presents a great potential for researches. Although there have been many recent studies on autism, there is a gap in what concerns language and communication. So far, emphasis has been on aspects of social interaction, diagnostic and prevalence.

It is widely known that there are certain deficits in communication, such as, the absence of expressive body cues (in non-verbal communication), deficits in understanding colloquial exchanges, and speech that is not adjusted the context (in verbal communication). Several elements in the speech of a subject with autism account for it being regarded as strange, unproductive, monotonous and unusual, such as a) the difficulty in using pronouns properly, particularly, with pronoun inversions; b) the repetition of questions which have already been answered or of fixed sentences in a mediated echolalic process; c) the literal understanding of metaphors or idiomatic slangs; and, d) the difficulty in using predicative abbreviations[4] [9].

In a study involving with neurotypical, mentally impaired and children with autism, the kind of gestures children use to communicate have been analyzed [10] and three main categories of gestures emerged: deictic (pointing); instrumental, to organize others' behavior; and, expressive, to share emotions. The study reveals that while typical and mentally impaired children use the three types of gestures, the group of children with autism only uses deictic

4 Predicative abbreviations consist of replacind the subject of a sentence so that the predicative remains as a hidden subject. For example: "Laura always buys bread at the grocery at the corner. She takes a bag and some change her mother leaves on the fridge." The second statement has a predicative abbreviation. It contains the action and the subject is implicit (WERTSCH, 1988).

and instrumental gestures. Besides that, other studies have established that children with autism face difficulties when it comes to using time and space pragmatic markers [11, 12], expressing mental states [13, 14], using adequate expressions and gestures [15], organizing more complex and "if-so" statements [16].

As for stories and narratives, the greatest difficulty for children with autism seems to lie in the ability to follow a narrative with multiple characters and organize each character's specific traits and personality. It is also hard for them to follow a character's way of thinking and to put themselves into the character's position [9, 10, 17, 18].

Such deficits in symbolization affect communication because it requires an active use of symbols for representation, especially, when situations involve more abstract elements such as feelings and emotions. Narratives demand the narrator to organize information for a potential listener and to select relevant aspects from the listener's perspective. Researchers have tried to explain such deficits for understanding narratives through the Theory of Mind [11, 13, 14, 16, 19, 20]. In those researches, it is hypothesized that people with autism fail to read other people's state of minds and understand their intentions, beliefs and emotions.

From another perspective, problems in communication could be associated with joint attention [1] or mutual imitation [21]. A recent research, consistent with previous studies, has focused adults diagnosed with high functioning autism or Asperger's syndrome [22]. It has not found deviation in phonology and syntax or deficits in the subjects' ability to understand and extract the plot of narratives. There was significant difference in the use of referents, though. As a consequence, narratives have been less coherent and less organized. Just as in [9], the research has identified pronominal inconsistencies, preference for simple and unbound sentences, disregard for the relationship of a specific event with what happened previously, and limited use of time expressions.

In another research [22], however, subjects are able to apprehend the structure of the story and follow the main plot as they mention all the relevant events of the narrative. Such outcome confirms that adults diagnosed with high functioning autism or Asperger's syndrome do not present difficulties with morphosyntactic aspects but rather a limited perception of a character's intentions and inner states in the story, that is, in pragmatics of communication.

Other study, aiming at the identification of the symbolic understanding of images with three children aged 7 to 9 years old [23], has shown it is possible to use functional communication successfully. In that study, non-verbal children not employing any type of visual/symbolic communication previously have undergone a process of systematic visual literacy consisting of understanding family, people, actions and sequences. Each category has been composed by a set of 10 symbols (or photographs); and, after nine weeks the proposal of intervention has shown positive results as children begin using the images to communicate requests, define tasks and other communicative activities. Such research adds to other of the kind focusing functional communication in autism [24].

Functional communication has started in the 90s with the Picture Exchange Communication System (PECS). PECS is an Alternative Communication (AC) system with a behavioral methodology for children with social communication deficits. Its main goal is to teach functional communication by means of hierarchical organization, basic principles of behavior such as modeling, differential reinforcement, stimulus control, control transference of stimulus through delayed strategies of questions [23].

PECS is one of several psychoeducational programs for people with autism available nowadays [25]. It seeks to stimulate spontaneous communication through potential reinforcers, images and physical exchanges. The system is organized into six hierarchical phases interwined with a method of behavior analysis and teaching. Although PECS seems functionally efficient, our critique is targeted at the strong behavioral control imposed by the system and its disregard for prerequisite abilities for language use, such as joint attention, imitation or visual contact as previously discussed.

Summing up, it is important to note that even children with autism who do not evidence language impairment might benefit from communication support systems at times, as a way to compensate for their lack of understanding of language semantics or pragmatics [26]. Is such cases, where speech is not present, the use of alternative communication systems can promote and develop processes to facilitate communication (facilitated communication). This way, the use of technology may contribute to the sociocognitive development of those subjects [27]; and, alternative communication systems may assist them in developing meaningful communication [9, 17, 23].

3. Alternative communication: Methodology and resource in an approach to autism

Alternative communication (AC) in one of the most important areas within the field known as Assistive Technology. It encompasses technical aids for communication, be it to complement, supplement or provide alternatives to make the communicative process happen.

There are several systems of AC. These provide a vast repertoire of representative elements, such as photographs, drawings and pictograms. Support for those systems may require either low (concrete material) or high (computational systems) technological devices. The importance of AC lies in the communicative strategies and techniques to promote subjects' autonomy for communicative instances so; it is secondary whether support is mediatic or not.

Given the impact language development on human development, subjects presenting deficits in communication can benefit from the use of AC systems as application of techniques and technology go beyond its instrumental character to enhance the development of abilities to use linguistic symbols intentionally. Considering that in the case of autism, communication deficits may exhibit alterations in language use, form or content in pragmatic level, and to a lesser extent, in syntactic, morphosyntactic, phonological or phonetic level, the importance of employing an AC system is more concerned with adequate reception and production processes, and those play an inter-related role [28].

Although the use of AC dates from the 90s, researches are recent. One of the first works was the adaptation and standardization of the PECS [29, 30]. It is also worthy of note the research on language development and meaning construction supported by AC with three children with autism [31], which revealed relevant outcomes.

More recent studies [32, 33, 34, 35] have involved the use of AC with Global Development Disorders (autism and Cornelia-Lange's syndrome). Those studies have also come to important results, particularly, when AC processes are supported by digital technologies.

According to the studies cited above, there is significant improvement in communication processes both in enunciation and pragmatics for subjects with autism when an AC system acts as tool of mediation between subjects in interaction. We believe that when AC is adapted to the needs of subjects with autism, it serves as a factor of facilitation and proximity because it contributes with an alternative for communication and establishes a "bridge" between people.

AC systems may function as bridge for human communication. However, it cannot be naively assumed that a technological support can stand on its own. On the contrary, an AC resource must be clearly founded on a methodology epistemologically grounded. The AC system presented in the following session (SCALA) is constituted of technological, human and social elements which are interwined to build an integral relationship, as highlighted by a researcher when stating that "[...] *more important than [...] any resource to intermediate dialogue, it is time, attention to listen and dedication granted to one another*" [36] (p. 139).

Two versions of SCALA have been developed by our team: web and tablet. Development has started in 2009 and the version for tablets is currently undergoing experimentation in a study with three children aged 4 diagnosed with autism.

4. Technology and autism: SCALA project

Researches on the use of technological applications for subjects with autism is frequent in the literature. One of the first studies involving technology and autism used computer-aided instruction (CAI) to stimulate the language development of children with autism [37]. Other studies have been published reporting the positive effects of technological applications in the process of teaching how to read and write [38, 39, 44], problem-solving [40, 41], social interaction [27, 42], and, cognition and learning [27, 39, 43].

Improvement of language use and children's learning how to read and write have been reported by [38] and [44]. In Brazil, the first study dates from 1975 [45]. It has been developed in the Laboratory of Artificial Intelligence of Edinburgh with a seven-year-old child with autism, with the use of Logo[5]. It has pointed out the use of Logo facilitated the process of interaction of the child with other people because "[...] the turtle assumed the role of mediator in the interaction of D. with other people and served as an object to help the development of mental schemes [...]" [45] (p. 73).

5 LOGO is a computational tool in which a student controls an icon represented by a turtle through simple commands. Designed by Seymour Papert in the 70s, it was the first computational tool especially projected to be constructivist and grounded on Genetic Epistemology.

Other positive outcomes of the studies above include gains in communication and motivation. Such correlations are often observed in a structured and communicative environment supported by technology and organized for interventions with subjects with autism [27]. Even when more guided [38] or more flexible [45] softwares are employed, results are productive. Such outcome could be traced back to the pedagogical strategy adopted by the teacher, who acts as a more experienced partner because the use of computers, particularly in virtual learning environments designed to adapt to the subject's interests and needs, becomes relevant and important tools of mediation as advocated under a sociohistorical conception [3].

Once strategies are added to the flexibility, adaptation and complexification processes inherent to digital technologies, they help to promote sociocognitive development of participants. Nevertheless, it is necessary to establish strategies for different learning environments, learning situations and subjects in interaction so that the introduction of technology can contribute with its qualitative differential for the enhancement of social interaction of subjects with autism [46]. In doing so, researches corroborate that the use of technologies can help people with autism communicate and interact [47].

Mobile devices also represent a possibility for the use of applications to assist users as well. Their utility extends into day by day activities as they are easy to handle, can be used in different places and allow connectivity to other devices. Connectivity in particular can be quite useful to enable communication and learning in groups and, as a consequence, can help foster the integration of subjects in their social environment [48].

On sociability, a recent study with high functioning autism and Asperger's syndrome adults users of online social networks has found that the structuring features of computer-mediated communication (CMC) help and promote their participation in social interactional processes [49]. Similar results have been identified in a study focusing chat room interaction [27]. In addition, a research by [50] highlights that engagement in mediated communication may not only foster participation, but also enhance learning of social rules of turn taking and dialog maintenance when supported by intelligent computational systems. Despite the likely advantages of CMC, it is important to consider its potential limitations and complications when it intensifies problems associated with trust, secrecy, inflexibility and perspectivation [51].

Turn-taking, which underlies unstructured social talk, poses a challenge which can be even greater if some sensorial hypersensibility (to lights, sounds, smell and touch) is associated with the syndrome. In those cases, communication controlled by a computational device may play a role in the maintenance of social relationship and management of feelings of loneliness and depression [52].

Adults with Asperger's may reveal intense isolation and difficulties to initiate social interaction [53]. They often lack a model of behavior socially acceptable and, as a result, may behave in a way that impacts their communication with other people negatively. Hence, alternative means of communication, like CMC, and other platforms easily available such as Orkut, Facebook, and other social networks, can be useful for the promotion of interaction of people with autism [27, 49, 50].

CMC offers users with autism control over their environment as well as over problems with prosody and intonation [49]. A study developed by e-mail with adults with Asperger's Syndrome has found that visual anonymity, time flexibility and the permanence allowed by the internet help diminish the social and emotional pressures of interpersonal communication as well as the cognitive complexity of the processes involved [49]. In particular, the authors state that online communities provide a space for interchanges and talks for people with similar interests or problems, so people with autism do benefit from those possibilities and structuring characteristics of CMC. In their study, 16 adults with high functioning autism or Asperger's syndrome have been interviewed on their daily activities and participation in social networks and attested that CMC tends to be beneficial for the initiation of social interactions – more than half of the interviewees participated in some type of social network. However, limitations and drawbacks in the interactions in social networks have been reported as well, which often refer to initiation of contact, maintenance of interaction for long periods and issues of security and trust. As a result, those users seek to interact with people already known from other spaces[6].

In spite of the benefits reported in studies, few address AC in technological systems with non-verbal subjects with autism. We know that communication with subjects with autism can resemble the "Tower of Babel" and challenges are greater when subjects are non-verbal[7]. In this case, we are in a rather complex situation which requires the adoption of strategies and resources to "climb up the tower". In the researches presented here, we notice that the use of technology is promising for the processes of communication and interaction. That brings us to some important questions: is it possible to identify the same benefits when allying the potential of CMC with AC? And, if so, how to use AC with mobile devices with non-verbal children with autism?

In this specific research node (AC, technology and autism), there are few studies on mobile devices for AC that focus people with the syndrome. In the literature review, in addition to the work of our research group, we found a research with the system Sc@ut [47]. Sc@ut is an AC system adapted to be a communicator for Pocket PC and Nintendo DS. According to the authors, the use of the system in groups of children with autism has shown an improvement in the behavior of subjects in oral language. With some subjects, the models of communication provided by the system were used to train social skills and daily life activities[8] [48]. The studies developed by our research group are reported in the following session.

6 This is typical within other social groups investigated. In general, confidence is stronger and more consistent among stigmatized group minorities [54].

7 Researches point out that a third of children with autism are non-verbal. Such proportion fells to 14 to 20% when they receive early intervention [55].

8 Another product under development by [47] is a platform for the creation of pedagogic activities for Ipad and Iphone. Activities are diverse including navigation, association, memory games, puzzles, sequencing, visual and aural perception, vocabulary, visuo-spatial coordination, among others. However, this product (Picaa) has not been tested with children with autism yet.

5. Development centered in contexts of use

Since 2009, when we started the development of SCALA, we have aimed at supporting language development of children with autism presenting deficits in communication. The epistemological basis of the sociohistorical theory, which we adopt, implies a conceptual re-organization of the software development process known as User-Centered Design (UCD). In UCD, the objective goes beyond subject-object interaction and focuses on designing strategies to allow interaction and communication between children with autism and other interlocutors [32, 34, 56]. SCALA is composed of three modules: board, narratives and free communication and follows a UCD approach.

From a sociohistorical perspective and the theoretical premises already presented, our approach not only contemplates the subject with disabilities, but that subject in interaction, which broadens our focus of investigation to (a) the **social contexts** in which (b) **cultural practices** of communication and literacy are developed by (c) **different participants** through (d) **mediating actions**.

The general guidelines of the UCD consider the macro context of human development in social interaction as the basis for the analysis of cases. Characteristics and needs of individuals cannot be understood apart from the contexts in which they belong. As a consequence, the development of assistive technology goes beyond a functional view of the human being. In spite of so, we do not ignore functional aspects in our proposal, we consider them within the cultural spectrum in which the AC is to operate. Each individual "inhabits" many contexts in which is more or less active in face of different cultural practices. In some cases, those practices happen within a triadic mediated action (individual-mediator-object) which entails learning and development. So, our focus of analysis is always the individual in relation with his/her different contexts. On its turn, each context impacts our relationships, consequently, the mediations that are possible. In time, we do not regard the cultural context as something that limits the individual, but as an element that shapes the relationship. This is why it is of importance to consider social contexts in the development of technology that will be employed as a qualitative resource and psychological tool in the mediating action.

Context, under such conception, exceeds the notion of physical space. It constitutes a condition that represents the action and is crossed by a space-time dimension. This dimension includes not only physical space but social space, and four types of time: a) present, which is the microgenetic time, i.e., the time now, b) lived, which refers to human history, or the ontogenetic time c) historical, which refers to one's personal story and is related to culture; and, at last, d) future, which is a projection, what one imagines will happen, one's own expectations and that of others, the wishes, the intentions that projects oneself to the future. Those four times frames pervade contexts and are constantly updated, so, they must be taken into consideration when we project assistive technology systems.

The analysis of the different frames of time starts with the present one – microgenetic – and through it, the others are recovered. An ethnographic approach is central in that analysis because "informants" provides information about lived and historical time that allows us to project into the future [57]. As ethnographic research is strongly based on discourse, therefore, discourse itself is a powerful informant. Because discourse is imbued with subjectivity, a report of memories and expectations, it may be argued that it does not provide a wholly truthful account. However, as subjectivity is an important aspect within the sociohistorical research, triangulation of the data is adopted as a regulating mechanism [58].

The configuration of contexts underlies sociohistorical research. The nature of contexts is a discursive one, in which language emerges and allows us to analyze various elements: persons, situations, cultural practices and mediating actions within those practices (Figure 1) in relation to time. Thus, context cannot be regarded as a static element as it plays a role in the interaction too. Besides the agents (people) – subject A1, subject A2 –, overlapping contexts need to be included in the analysis of contexts of use.

The overview of contexts constitutes the macro level of investigation necessary to deepen the understanding of the phenomenon of communication within educational spaces. In the micro level, triads (subject-mediator, non-verbal subject and mediating actions) represent the starting point for the understanding of the processes of mediation with technologies. Such methodological perspective supports the development of technological resources (for instance, SCALA) in a differentiated way, that is, different from traditional processes of development and different from processes based on UCD, which involve users in the process of development and take their needs, expectations and experiences into consideration.

In SCALA, there is not a single model of user but a diverse range of agents involved with many peculiarities that differ in expectations and experiences, this is why we propose a broader view. We are not only interested in the user, as in the UCD, but in the peculiarities and specificities of the various agents in interaction as well. Our focus encompasses the action implied in the interaction, the cultural practices in which agents and technological resources are embedded.

Besides UCD, another proposal is the Activity-Centered Design (ACD). ACD focuses the activity that is performed and, as in the UCD, tries to create a model of activity. Considering that literacy practices cannot be thought of as an activity but as a set of practices that vary across different situations, we propose a Context-Centered Design (CCD). In this sort of development, differentiated sociohistorical contexts provide the guidelines to orient system development. In other words, what people do in different contexts, with different objectives and scenarios is what guides this project development. Figure 1 shows a scheme of CCD.

Three multi-case researches underlie SCALA developed. The first research allowed us to identify mediation strategies and validate the methodological proposal for intervention with communication with children with ASD [33]. The second case study was concerned with the interaction and intervention with a child aged 5-6 diagnosed with ASD and presenting deficits in communication. This case study was a follow-up to the previous one and derived strategies for the development of communication with the use of a first prototype in this phase [35]. Interventions allowed a broader understanding of the process of use implementation of AC with children with autism, and provided input on how a tool for such purpose should be developed.

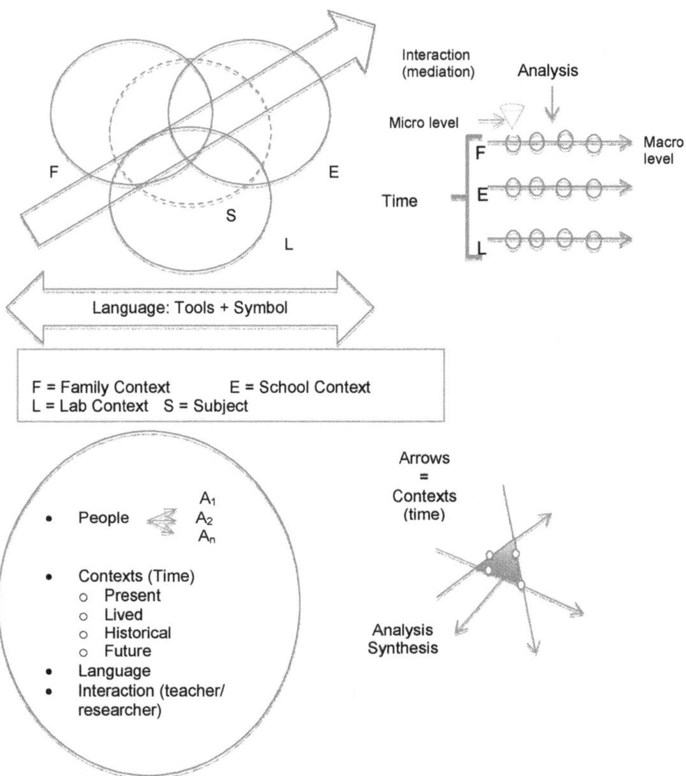

Figure 1. Scheme of Context-Centered Design (CCD)

Requirements, like touch screens and the adaptation of the size of the figures among other aspects, have significantly contributed to the second version of SCALA. A new version, now considering mobile devices and fast connection with the internet is under development (2011-2012) and has been informed by the third study, currently involving three subjects from three different cultural contexts. From the family context, the study took into consideration daily interactions, hygiene, leisure time, among other information. Besides family, other contexts include school and laboratory. The proposal of the controlled context is to investigate interaction with peers by inserting 3 children with autism in the same social space and at present time.

As it is possible to observe, development and investigation imbricate in a spiral process where each process repeats itself reaching greater complexity, and thus, improving the system which proceeds development according to the principles of CCD. To develop SCALA, on the one hand, we address the needs of communication of non-verbal children, the expectations of their teachers as mediators of educative practices and count on the intense participation of family to use and adapt those strategies and resources [32, 34, 59, 60]. On the other hand, research trajectory involves several investigation projects developed by the research group in different spaces and moments, with points of intersection and team consolidation through regular meetings to keep investigation on track. Spiral development starts from a deep analysis of existing systems[9] adding to the results of the multi-case researches, which gradually informs the construction of requirements for the system and is constantly adjusted.

From a technological standpoint SCALA has as its main features, a module for building communication boards, a module for the construction of stories, and a module for free communication. It also encompasses common application features such as the ability to import files, edit sounds, save, export, and manage the various files generated by the system (Figure 2). The menu on the left to the user presents the categories of images that can be used with all the three modules and the horizontal menu bar displays the features.

From a predefined layout one can fill each card by clicking on the categories of images. Each image has a caption pattern which can be edited. For each card it is possible to record sounds and hear them. If the user does not want to record a sound, a speech synthesizer will read the caption (otherwise, the sound recorded by the user will be supplied).

In addition to the existing images in the system, it is possible to add personal images allowing customization and adaptation to the sociohistorical context of the user. Finally, the last feature designed was the animation of actions. This feature was introduced as empirical studies have shown evidence that animated actions may be more suitable to forge understanding of metaphorical and symbolic elements with autism [46, 61, 62].

SCALA is currently available for two platforms (web e android), which allows its use with mobile devices. In the next session, some preliminary results are presented.

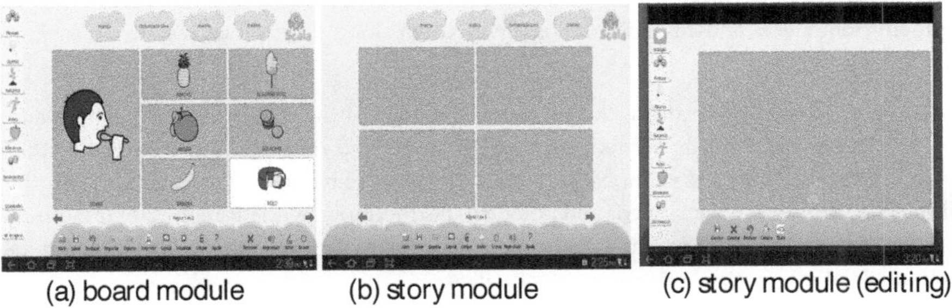

Figure 2. Board and Story modules in the version for Android for tablets

9 The main softwares available in the market have been explored, for example, Amplisoft, Boardmaker,and other free systems whose traits concerning interaction and narrative building were relevant to think about the system's requirements. A complete synthesis of such assessment was developed by [35] as part of her masters research.

6. Development and preliminary results

In the session, an extract of some preliminary results of our research is presented. It comprises the period of time raging from August 2011 to May 2012. The subjects are three non-verbal children diagnosed with autism aged 4 years old. Three contexts have been taken into account: family, school and laboratory, but, in this report, we mainly focus on the interactions in the context of the laboratory, so, just a few considerations about other contexts are referred.

Interactions have been planned upon the methodology of mediating actions, with particular focus on the promotion of scenes of joint attention in order to accomplish communication and social interaction of the subjects involved. Those interactions happened simultaneously with the three subjects once a week in the laboratory. Interactions in the laboratory took place weekly and duration was flexible in the beginning[10] to adapt to the needs of individuals. In addition, there were visits to each subject's home and school followed by observation and initial guidance to mothers and school personnel. This way, the subjects' contexts encompassing greater social experiences and participation were accessed. The first contact was with the mothers, school and teachers with the distribution of some instruments for data collection[11] to help set up an initial profile of the subjects.

The interventions of the researcher in the three contexts do not follow a linear fashion. Visits are scheduled according to opportunity and the needs identified in the course of the research. Interventions are filmed for later analysis and to subsidize reconstruction and development of new possibilities of interactional arrangements so as to contribute to subjects' development across contexts.

Besides the scenes of joint attention, which have been promoted as part of the methodology of intervention, subjects had the opportunity to interact with physical AC materials as instruments of mediation of those scenes. Then, during the first weeks, AC material employing both low and high technology was used along with other resources, as Presented in the figure 3.

Mediating actions had a focus on the triadic interactions of the mediator with subjects and objects acting as instruments of mediation to further expand the interactions with the other subjects. With the first interventions in the lab, it was possible to establish bonds with the children and get to know their needs and potential. Furthermore, with the help of their mothers and school teachers, it was possible to outline a descriptive profile of their forms of communication, social interaction and initial potentialities.

In spite of the same diagnosis, the three children have very distinctive characteristics within the symptoms of the syndrome and are accompanied by diverse professionals in therapeutic interventions. They are referred to as Case 1, 2 and 3 in the table 1.

10 In the beginning, meetings were shorter and gradually increased in time.

11 Open interviews, anamnesis and consent forms

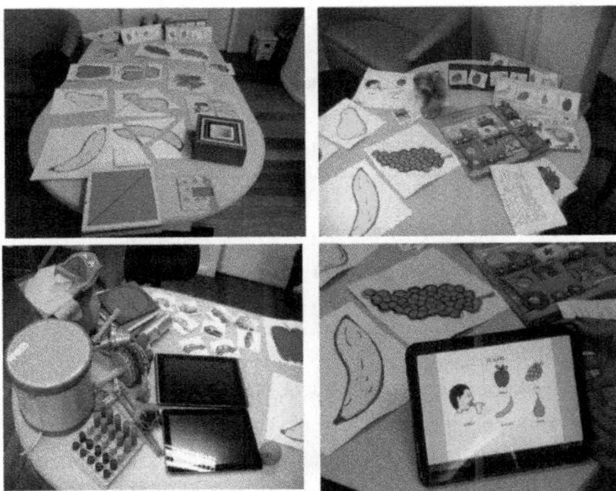

Figure 3. Example of AC material of low and high technology

Case 1	Boy, 3.10 y.o., living with his parents and two older sisters; attends nursery (level 3) school in the afternoon. Some abnormality in his development was noticed at the age of 1.3 y. o. as he did not show any vocabulary. ASD was diagnosed at the age of 1.9 by a team of professionals (pediatrician, neuropsychologist and a psychiatrist).
Communication	Makes some sounds, makes meaningful facial expressions (looks) to pay attention, when he is called, to get to know the environment and closes his eyes in protest. He smiles to demonstrate satisfaction and joy and cries, grumbles and mumbles to show contrariety. Body expressions involve pointing and touching what he wants with his finger and waving. Is starting AC with speech therapist. Communicates spontaneously through gestures in order to have his wishes realized. Does not present stereotyped behavior.
Social interaction and understanding	Accepts touch. Understands the meaning of the objects and his own existence. Demonstrates understanding of other people without engaging in turn taking. Interacts when is requested to by sitting at a table. Can interact with objects and other people for short or medium periods of time.
Potencialities – preferences	Can deal with changes in routine. Does not react contradictorily in the presence of people who are strange to him. Is fascinated by lights, fans, drains and objects that spin. Appreciates looking at the mirror. Use communicative gestures through meaningful facial and bodily expressions. Can hold a pencil, paints with some limitation, scribbles. Uses his index finger to point at things he wants. Can eat with independence and can put on shoes without shoelaces.

Case 1	Boy, 3.10 y.o., living with his parents and two older sisters; attends nursery (level 3) school in the afternoon. Some abnormality in his development was noticed at the age of 1.3 y. o. as he did not show any vocabulary. ASD was diagnosed at the age of 1.9 by a team of professionals (pediatrician, neuropsychologist and a psychiatrist).
	Is in the process of toilet training and learning to dress and undress with independence.
Case 2	Boy, 4.2 y.o. lives with parents and a brother. Some abnormality in his development was noticed at the age of 2.3 y.o.. ASD was diagnosed at the age of 2.3 by a neuropediatrician and psychologist. Attends nursery school in the afternoon.
Communication	Presents some language delay. It is difficult to understand what he says. Uses a proper language. Understands speech but does not engage in turn taking. Facial expressions are observed when he is upset, cries and grumbles to show contrariety. Does not sustain visual contact. Knocks his head to call attention or squeezes his arms and legs. Moves his hands and fingers in a strange way. To get what he wants, uses other people's arm or hand. Pointing is not part of his routine. Has difficulty in sitting still or remaining in an activity. Likes to scribbles, but with no apparent meaning. Does not use any form of alternative communication.
Social interaction and understanding	Resists to be touched. Contact is accepted only by family members. Limited understanding of the meanings of objects or people. Does not get attached to his environment or shows a sense of belonging. Interaction is restricted to objects when they are interesting to him and gets attached to them.
Potencialities – preferences	Appreciates music, fascination for lights, mirrors and bright eyes. Hyposensitive in relation to senses, laughs for no apparent reason, shows good coordination. Likes to jump, lie on the floor and run. Food compulsiveness needs to be managed. Depends on other people to dress, undress and for hygiene.
Case 3	Boy, 3.5 y.o. lives with parents. Some abnormality in his development was noticed at the age of 1.3 y.o.., neurologist attested ASD. Uses anti-psychotic (Resperidal) and anti-convulsive medication. Attends nursery school in the afternoon..
Communication	Oral communication is expressed through few grumbles. Communicates through gestures with people who are familiar to him. To get what he wants, uses other people's arm or hand. Does not point at objects. Facial expressions are observed when he is displeased, cries and grumbles to show contrariety. Frustration is expressed through aggression (beating himself and others, pulling one's hair, bites). Shows great difficulty in demonstrating what he wants to communicate. Does not use any form of alternative communication.

Case 1	Boy, 3.10 y.o., living with his parents and two older sisters; attends nursery (level 3) school in the afternoon. Some abnormality in his development was noticed at the age of 1.3 y. o. as he did not show any vocabulary. ASD was diagnosed at the age of 1.9 by a team of professionals (pediatrician, neuropsychologist and a psychiatrist).
Social interaction and understanding	Does not accept physical contact and does not make eye contact. Elects small spaces to stay. In some moments, he seems to "unplug" and becomes apathetic to everything and everyone Does not accept the mediation of the researcher and in rare moments, it happens with some object he is interested in.
Potencialities – preferences	Loud noises call his attention, shows fascination for lights, interest in small details of objects. Keeps a fixed and strange look at his fingers and hands. Often puts objects in his mouth. Faces difficulty to run, jump, climb and go down the stairs. Exaggerated attachment and attraction to certain objects, likes to spin them and does not use games properly. Changes in routine are not well accepted. Sometimes he is too active and other times too passive. Is afraid of wide spaces and symmetric floor.

Table 1. Initial profile of communication, social interaction and potentialities of subjects.

As can be noticed, only one of the subjects used the pointing function. Due to that, initial sessions focused on actions to make that gesture meaningful. SCALA software was used in two versions with symbols and boards with tablets. In the beginning, there was a great need to associate concrete material with the symbols in the boards and, afterwards, the gesture of pointing emerged with the fascination for the tablet technology.

The subject from case 2 accepts to be touched and soon learns to point. He also increases lateral visual contact. Although we accomplished only a few instances of mediation, he started interacting with the technological tool and increased attention span through the observation of details. On its turn, subject 1 improves pointing and eye contact and starts participating in scenes of joint attention in response to the employed mediating actions (mediator-subject-object). He soon shows great autonomy in dealing with the tablet. At last, subject 3 required more time to accept some physical contact and to fix his eyes on the activities proposed. Pointing was initially motivated by the sound produced by this touch on the screen.

Together with SCALA, several free applications have been tried with the children (Figure 4). Applications were picked according to the profile of each of the subjects and that was important to promote the appropriation and understanding of the technology, as seen in Figure 5, along with the use of AC boards (Figure 6).

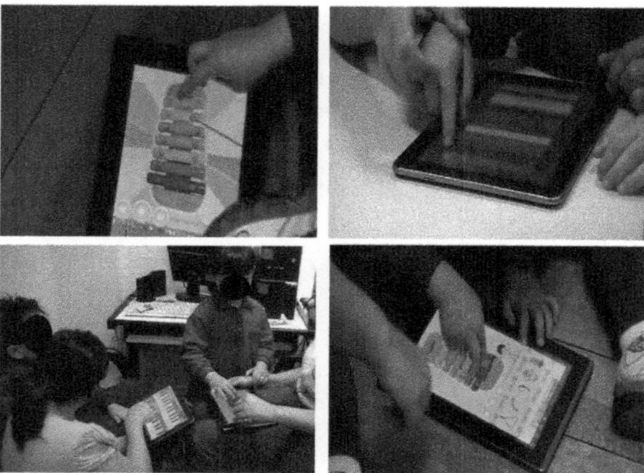

Figure 4. Using different *tablet* applications

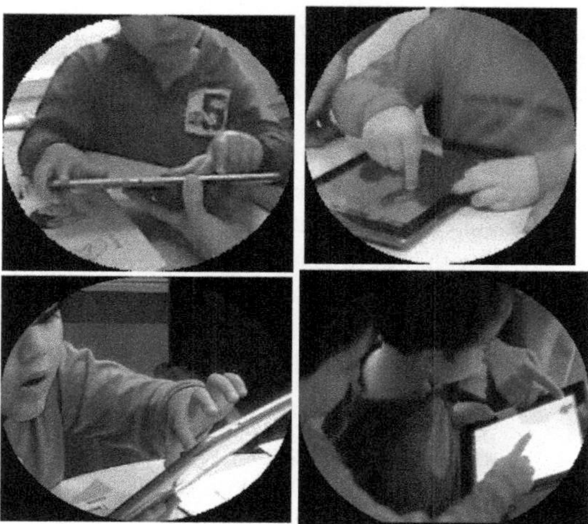

Figure 5. Using *tablets* with subjects with autism

With the use of tablets, we could notice attention spans increased for all the subjects. Speech was also prompted in all mediations. So, subjects' range of vocabulary has increased. Subject 1 showed easiness with the technology and the participation as an intentional agent in mediated actions. He is currently producing more words with two syllables and participating in scenes of joint attention in the mediations with other subjects.

Although subject 2 demonstrates he prefers to interact with the equipment on his own, he also starts participating in scenes of joint attention in the mediated actions. In some few instances, he initiates interactions with the other subjects spontaneously. It is possible to notice the verbalization of some isolated words and that he accepts being touched and demonstrates affection through hugs and kisses.

Subject 3, through mediating actions accepts touch and demonstrates affection through kisses and hugs. Aggression is only expressed when he feels some pain. His interactions with the object increase and he starts participating in some mediating actions with the researcher. Only one word was said after great insistence, but the symbols of alternative communication start being understood, which is likely to contribute to his way of communication soon.

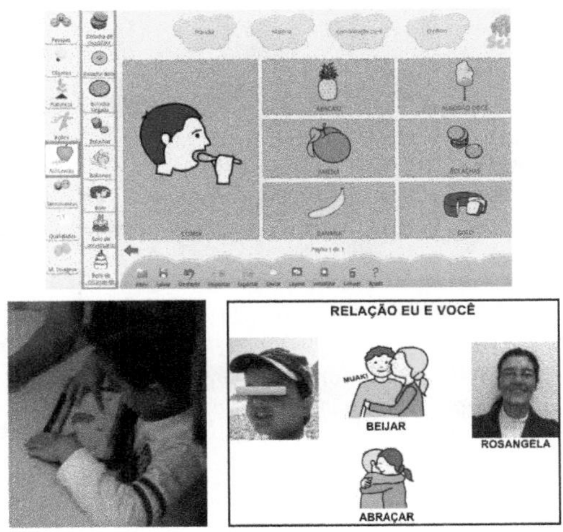

Figure 6. the use of SCALA with subjects with autism in the tablet and a board with symbols

The first image of Figure 3 shows one of the subjects interacting with AC software – SCALA. The second shows a board constructed with the software and meant to be used in the mediated actions. The third image is a board adopting low-technology with printed material.

Apart from the work in the laboratory, mothers were asked to use alternative communication at home. As needs came up, mothers turned to us and together we constructed boards. A tablet was purchased by two families (subjects 1 and 2), so the children started using it in family contexts too. As for schools, the teachers of subjects 1 and 2 have requested some boards to use in that environment too, but we perceived a lack of understanding about how to integrate AC in the school context. Therefore, we are providing two training courses, for teachers and assistants and for the school team.

The results referred here are preliminary as the project stretches until 2013. However, they are consistent with previous research [27, 33, 50, 63] showing relevant outcomes for the social and cognitive development of subjects with autism through the use of digital learning environment as instruments of mediation. Just as the present study, they have also adopted a sociohistorical view where mediating actions widen the level of development through the use of symbols and tools in a way that the zone of proximal development is adjusted until internalization of concepts is complete.

In fact, we can consider the significant improvement in both social interaction and cognitive development of subjects with autism with the introduction of technology from a sociohistorical perspective as it allows more flexible adaptive and abstraction processes with increasing levels of complexity.

7. Conclusion

To sum up, it is important to highlight that developing assistive technology for alternative communication as proposed in this chapter, that is with Context-Centered Design, implicates a multidimensional process involving technological innovations, pedagogic mediation, cultural practices and contexts, as well as, specific formations pervaded by critical analysis to favor the creation of new technologies with differentiated theoretical and methodological proposals.

The introduction of alternative communication can go far beyond the specialized spaces in the scope of Health and Education, such as the rooms of multifunctional resources[12], for instance. For those who need it, alternative communication is a tool to be used in varied social spaces and systematically in daily life.

Acknowledgements

We would like to thank

- CAPES (Coordination for higher Education Staff Development), which through PROESP (Special Education Support Program), has funded graduate students involved in this project;
- CNPq (National Counsel of Technological and Scientific Development) for research scholarships to undergraduate students and grants to research professors;
- FAPERGS (Foundation of Research Support of Rio Grande do Sul) for the financial support through through the Edict Pesquisador Gaúcho 2009 that funded the development of phases II and III of SCALA Project; and

12 Rooms of multifunctional resources are equipped with diverse assistive technologies applications that are distributed by the Ministry of Education to regular public schools that serve students with disabilities or special needs through a specialized educational support outside school hours.

- PROPESQ/UFRGS (Research Dean Office of Federal University of Rio Grande do Sul) for the infrastructure and financial support to SCALA project.

Project funded by CAPES and FAPERGS. Article developed from researches funded by CAPES (PROESP program), CNPq (Grant for Productivity in Technological Development and Innovative Extension) and FAPERGS ("Gaucho" Researcher Edict 2010).

Author details

Liliana Maria Passerino[1] and Maria Rosangela Bez[2]

*Address all correspondence to: liliana@cinted.ufrgs.br

1 Graduate Program in Education (PPGEDU) and Computer Science and Education (PGIE) and the Interdisciplinary Center of Technologies in Education - CINTED/UFRGS, Computer Science and Education, Brazil

2 Interdisciplinary Center of Technologies in Education - CINTED/UFRGS, Brazil

References

[1] Tomasello, M. Origens culturais da aquisição do conhecimento humano. São Paulo: Martins Fontes, 2003.

[2] Vygotsky, L. S. A Construção do Pensamento e da Linguagem (texto integral traduzido do russo). São Paulo: Martins Fontes, 2001.

[3] Vygotsky, L. S. Formação Social da Mente. 6.ed.- São Paulo: Martins Fontes, 1988.

[4] Tomasello, M; Carpenter, M. The Emergence of Social Cognition in Three Young Chimpanzees. Monogr Soc Res Child Dev. 2005;70(1):vii-132.

[5] Wertsch, J. Vygotsky y la formación social de la mente. Serie Cognición y desarrollo humano. Barcelona: Ed. Paidós, 1988.

[6] Wertsch,J. La Mente en Acción. Buenos Aires: Aique, 1999.

[7] Wing, L. El Autismo en niños y adultos: Una guía para la família. Buenos Aires. Argentina: Paidós, 1998.

[8] Rivière, A. Colección Estructura y Procesos. Serie Pensamiento, Psicopatologia y Psiquiatría. Madrid, 2001.

[9] Jordan, R. & Powell, S. Understanding and Teaching Children with Autism. West Sussex, England: John Wiley&Sons, 1995.

[10] Peeters, T. Autism: From Theoretical Understanding to Educational Intervention. Whurr Publishers, 1998.

[11] Bruner, J., & Feldman, C. Theory of mind and the problem of autism. In S. Baron-Cohen, H. Tager-Flsberg & D. Cohen (Eds.), Understanding other minds: Perspectives from autism. Oxford: Oxford University Press, 1993.

[12] Loveland, K. & Tunali, B. Narrative language in autism and the theory of mind hypothesis: A wider perspective. In S. Baron-Cohen, H. Tager-Flusberg, and D. Cohen (Eds.), Understanding other minds: Perspectives from autism, pp. 247-266, Oxford University Press, 1993.

[13] Baron-Cohen, S. Without a theory of mind one cannot participate in a conversation. Cognition, 1988b, 29, 83–84.

[14] Baron-Cohen, S. Autismo: uma alteração cognitiva específica de "cegueira mental". Revista Portuguesa de Pedagogia, Ano XXIV, 1990, p.407-430.

[15] Loveland, K. A., Mcevoy, R. E., Tunali, B., & Kelley, M. L. Narrative story telling in autism and Down's syndrome. British Journal of Developmental Psychology, 1990, 8, 9–23.

[16] Tager-Flusberg, H., & Sullivan, K. Attributing mental states to story characters: A comparison of narratives produced by autistic and mentally retarded individuals. Applied Psycholinguistics, 1995, 16, 241–256.

[17] Sigman, M. & Capps, L. Niños y Niñas autistas. Série Bruner. Madrid: Morata, 2000.

[18] Hobson, P.R. El autismo y el desarrollo de la Mente. Madrid: Alianza Editorial, 1993.

[19] Baron-Cohen, S. Perceptual role taking and protodeclarative pointing in autism. British Journal of Developmental Psychology, 1989, 7, 113–127.

[20] Happé, F. An advance test of theory of mind: understanding of story characters' thoughts and feeling by able autistic, mentally handicapped, and normal children and adults. Journal f Autism and Development Disorders, 1994, 24, 129–154.

[21] Meltzoff, A. N., & Gopnik, A. (1993). The role of imitation in understanding persons and developing a theory of mind. In: S. Baron-Cohen, H. Tager-Flusberg, & D. J. Cohen (Eds), Understanding other minds. Oxford Medical Publications, 1993, p. 335–366.

[22] Colle, L.; Baron-Cohen, S.; Whellwrigth, S; van der Lely, H. Narrative Discourse in Adults with High-Functioning Autism or Asperger Syndrome. Journal Autism Dev Disord. 2008, 38:28–40 DOI 10.1007/s10803-007-0357-5.

[23] Cihak, D. Teaching students with autism to read pictures. Research in Autism Spectrum Disorders 1(2007) 318–329.

[24] Bondy, A., & Frost, L. The picture exchange communication system. Focus on Autistic Behavior, 1994, 9, 1–19.

[25] Bergeson, T.; Heuschel, M.; Harmon, B.; Gill, D.; Colwell, M.L. Los aspectos pedagógicos de los trastornos del espectro autista. Office of Superintendent of Public Instruction, (OSPI), 2003. Disponível on-line em: http://www.k12.wa.us.

[26] Bosa, C. Intervenções psicoeducacionais. Revista Brasileira de Psiquiatria. 2006;28(Supl I):S47-53.

[27] Passerino, L, M. & Santarosa, L. Autism and Digital Learning Environments: processes of interaction and mediation. Computers and Education, v. 51, p. 385-402, 2008.

[28] Passerino, L. M. A Comunicação Aumentativa e Alternativa no espaço do Atendimento Educacional Especializado: trajetórias imbricadas de investigação e desenvolvimento tecnológico. In: Anais VI Seminário Nacional de Pesquisa em Educação especial: Práticas Pedagógicas na educação Especial: multiplicidade do atendimento educacional especializado, 2011. v. 1. p. 1-17.

[29] Walter, C. A adaptação do sistema PECS de comunicação para o Brasil: uma comunicação alternativa para pessoas com autismo infantil. In: Marquezine MC, Almeida MA, Tanaka EDO, Mori N, Shimazaki, E., organizadores. Perspectivas multidiciplinares em educação especial. Londrina:Ed UEL. 1998. p.277-80.

[30] Walter, C. Os efeitos da adaptação do PECS associada ao Curriculum funcional em pessoas com autismo infantil [dissertação]. São Carlos (SP): Universidade Federal de São Carlos; 2000.

[31] Orrú, S. E. A constituição da linguagem de alunos autistas apoiada em Comunicação Suplementar Alternativa. Tese de Doutorado. Piracicaba: UNIMEP, 2006.

[32] Bez, M. R.; Passerino, L. M. Applying Alternative and Augmentative Communication to an inclusive group. In: WCCE 2009 - Education and Technology for a Better World Monday, 2009, Bento Gonçalves. WCCE 2009 Proceedings - Education and Technology for a Better World Monday. Germany : IFIP WCCE, 2009. v. 1. p. 164-174.

[33] Bez, M. R. Comunicação Aumentativa e Alternativa para sujeitos com Transtornos Globais do Desenvolvimento na promoção da expressão e intencionalidade por meio de Ações Mediadoras. Dissertação. Programa de Pós-Graduação em Educação - Faculdade de Educação. Universidade Federal Do Rio Grande Do Sul. Porto Alegre, 2010.

[34] Avila, B. G; Passerino, L. M. Comunicação Aumentativa e Alternativa e Autismo: desenvolvendo estratégias por meio do SCALA. In:Anais VI Seminário Nacional de Pesquisa em Educação especial: Práticas Pedagógicas na educação Especial: multiplicidade do atendimento educacional especializado, 2011. v. 1. p. 1-10

[35] Avila, B. G. Comunicação Aumentativa e Alternativa para o Desenvolvimento da Oralidade de Pessoas com Autismo. Dissertação de Mestrado. PPGEDU/UFRGS. 2011.

[36] Walter, C. O PECS adaptado no ensino regular: ma opção de comunicação alternativa para alunos com autismo. In: Nunes, L. Quiterio, P; Walter, C.; Schimer, C.;Braun, P.

(Org.) Comunicar é preciso: em busca das melhores práticas na educação do aluno com deficiência. Marilia: ABPEE, 2011 [192 p.] (p. 127-140).

[37] Colby, K. M. The Rationale for Computer-Based Treatment of Language Difficulties in Nonspeaking Autistic Children, Journal of Autism and Childhood Schizophrenia 1973, 3: 254–60.

[38] Heimann, M., Nelson, K.E., Tjus, T. & Gillberg, C. Increasing reading and communication skills in children with autism through an interactive multimedia computer program. Journal of Autism and Developmental Disorders, 1995, 25(5):459-80.

[39] Tjus, T.; Heimann, M. & Nelson, K. E. Gains in Literacy through the Use of a Specially Developed Multimedia Computer Strategy: Positive Findings from Thirteen Children with Autism, Autism 1998, 2: 139–56

[40] Jordan, R. & Powell, S. Improving Thinking in Autistic Children Using Computer Presented Activities. Communication, 1990, 24: 23–5.

[41] Jordan, R. & Powell, S. Teaching Autistic Children to Think More Effectively', Communication, 1990b, 24: Wiley&Sons, 1995.

[42] Parsons, S; Chell, P.; Leonard, A. Do adolescents with autistic spectrum disorders adhere to social conventions in virtual environments?. SAGE Publications and The National Autistic Society, 2005, Vol 9(1) 95–117.

[43] Bernard-Opiz, V.; Ross, K.; Tuttas, M.L. Computer assisted instruction for autistic children. Annals of the Academy of Medicine, 1990, v. 19, p. 611-616.

[44] Nelson, K. E., Heimann, M. & Tjus, T. Theoretical and Applied Insights from Multimedia Facilitation of Communication Skills in Children with Autism, Deaf Children, and Children with Other Disabilities. In: Adamson, L. & Romski, M. (eds) Communication and Language Acquisition: Discoveries from Atypical Development. Baltimore, MD: Brookes, 1997, p. 295-325.

[45] Valente, J. A. Informática na Educação Especial. In: VALENTE, J. A. (Org.) Liberando a Mente: Computadores na Educação Especial. Campinas, SP: Unicamp. 1991. 62-79.

[46] Passerino, L. M. Pessoas com autismo em ambientes digitais de aprendizagem : estudo dos processos de interação social e mediação. 2005. Universidade Federal do Rio Grande do Sul. Faculdade de Educação. Programa de Pós-Graduação em Informática na Educação. Disponível em http://hdl.handle.net/10183/13081.

[47] Rodríguez-Fórtiz, M. J., Fernández-Lopez, A., Rodriguez, M. L. Mobile Communication and Learning Applications for Autistic People. IN: Williams, Tim (Ed.) Autism Spectrum Disorders – From Genes to Environment. Rieka, Croatia: Intechweb.org, 2011 (p. 349-362).

[48] Rodríguez-Fórtiz, M. J., González, J. L., Fernández, A., Entrena, M., Hornos, M. J., Pérez, A., Carrillo, A. & Barragán, L. "Sc@ut: Developing Adapted Communicators for Special

Education". Procedia - Social and Behavioral Sciences, 2009, 1 (1), pp. 1348-1352. Elsevier.

[49] Burke, M. and Kraut, R. Mopping up: modeling wikipedia promotion decisions. Proc. CSCW ACM (2008), 27- 36.Colby, K. M. (1973). The Rationale for Computer-Based Treatment of Language Difficulties in Nonspeaking Autistic Children, Journal of Autism and Childhood Schizophrenia 3: 254–60

[50] Rabello , R. S.; Passerino, L. M.; Vicari, R. M.; Silveira, R. A. Interação e Autismo: Uso de Agentes Inteligentes para Detectar Déficits de Comunicação em Ambientes Síncronos. Revista Brasileira de Informática na Educação (2011) v. 19, n. 01.

[51] Seltzer, M.M., Krauss, M.W., Shattuck, P.T., Orsmond, G., Swe, A., & Lord, C. The Symptoms of Autism Spectrum Disorders in Adolescence and Adulthood. Journal of Autism and Developmental Disorders 33, 6 (2003), 565-581.

[52] Lainhart, J.E. and Folstein, S.E. Affective disorders in people with autism: a review of published cases. Journal of Autism and Developmental Disorders 24, 5 (1994), 587-601.

[53] Muller, E., Schuler, A., and Yates, G.B. Social challenges and supports from the perspective of individuals with Asperger syndrome and other autism spectrum disabilities. Autism, 2008, 12, 2, 173.

[54] Passerino, L & Montardo, S. P. Inclusão social via acessibilidade digital: proposta de inclusão digital para Pessoas com Necessidades Especiais (PNE). E-Compós (Brasília), 2007, v. 8, p. 1-18.

[55] Thunberg, G.; Ahlsén, E.; Sandberg, A. D. Autism, communication and use of a speech-generating device in different environments – a case study, Journal of Assistive Technologies, 2011, Vol. 5 Iss: 4, pp.181 - 198Tjus, T.;

[56] Passerino, L. M.; Avila, B. G.; Bez, M. R. SCALA: um Sistema de Comunicação Alternativa para o Letramento de Pessoas com Autismo. RENOTE. Revista Novas Tecnologias na Educação, v. 1, p. 1-10, 2010.

[57] Goetz, J. P. Etnography and qualitative design in educational research. Orlando, EUA: Academic Press, 1984.

[58] Yin, R. K. Case study research, design and methods, 3rd ed. Newbury Park: Sage Publications, 2003.

[59] Rodrigues, G. F. E se os outros puderem me entender? Os sentidos da Comunicação Alternativa e Suplementar produzidos por educadores especiais. 2011. Dissertação (mestrado) - Universidade Federal do Rio Grande do Sul. Faculdade de Educação. Programa de Pós-Graduação em Educação, Porto Alegre, BR-RS, 2011.

[60] Rodrigues, G. F.; Passerino, L. Formação permanente de professores e Comunicação Alternativa: uma aproximação necessária. In: I Seminário de Políticas Públicas de inclusão escolar no Rio Grande do Sul, 2010, Porto Alegre. Anais do I Seminário de Políticas Públicas de inclusão escolar no Rio Grande do Sul, 2010. p. 01-18.

[61] Barth, C; Passerino, L.M.; Santarosa, L. M. C. Descobrindo emoções: software para estudo da teoria da mente em sujeitos com autismo. CINTED. Porto Alegre, v.3, n.1, 2005. Disponível em: <http://www.cinted.ufrgs.br/>. Acesso em: 20 de mai. 2007.

[62] Barakova, E.; Gillessen, J.; Feijs, L. Social training of autistic children with interactive intelligent agents. Journal of Integrative Neuroscience, Vol. 8, No. 1 (2009) 23–34

[63] Bez, M. R. ; Passerino, L. M. Tecnologias Assistivas, salas de recursos e Inclusão escolar a partir da perspectiva sócio-histórica. In: VI Seminário Regional de Formação de gestores e Educadores do Programa Educação Inclusiva: Direito à Diversidade, 2010, Uruguaiana. VI Seminário Regional de Formação de gestores e Educadores do Programa Educação Inclusiva: Direito à Diversidade. Uruguaiana: Prefeitura Municipal de Uruguaiana, 2010. v. 1. p. 31-40.

Chapter 6

Early Intervention of Autism: A Case for Floor Time Approach

Rubina Lal and Rakhee Chhabria

Additional information is available at the end of the chapter

1. Introduction

Autism is a developmental disorder that affects a child's perception of the world and how the child learns from his or her experiences. Even among the most complex disabilities, autism remains an enigma. Autism is the frequently occurring form of a group of disorders known as Autism Spectrum Disorders (ASD). The term Autism Spectrum Disorders (ASD) covers diagnostic labels which include Autistic Disorder, High Functioning Autism, Asperger's Syndrome, and Pervasive Developmental Disorder – Not Otherwise Specified (PDD-NOS).

Autism Society of America [1] defines autism as a complex developmental disability that typically appears during the first three years of life and is the result of a neurological disorder that affects the normal functioning of the brain, impacting development in the areas of social interaction and communication skills. Autism has also been defined as a neurological disorder characterized by qualitative impairment in social interaction and communication as well as the presence of restricted, repetitive, and stereotyped patterns of behaviors, interests and activities [2]. Children with ASD share the social and communicative symptoms which are the core of autism, but they vary in severity of symptoms and in level of functioning.

The first three years of life are critical to a child's development. Parents take their child to the pediatrician, during this period for general health check up, screening and vaccinations. Although child with autism can be screened by 18 months by a pediatrician, parents often are the first ones to suspect behavioral deviations in their child. The mean age for such screening is approximately 15 months and in some cases it can be as early as 11 months [3]. According to the parents, children manifest patterns of extreme reactivity, either by getting upset when new stimulus is shown or by completely ignoring it. The infants often fail to copy verbal behavior of others and do not babble by 12 months.

Research reports a significant difference between age-matched infants with autism and typically developing infants with respect to visual attention to social stimuli, smile frequency, vocalization, object exploration engagement, facial expression, use of conventional gesture, and pointing to indicate interest [4].

Identifying autism in toddlers is a recent practice. A large number of children have been diagnosed reliably at 2 years. Professionals can now predict autism from the behaviors observed in a child younger than 2 years. Providing therapeutic intervention at this age would improve developmental and adaptive outcomes. The global trend in early intervention of autism is to provide training to parents so they can help the children develop in key areas of social responsiveness, attention skills, early communication skills, and interactive behavior.

2. Autism and social behavior

Difficulties in social relationships and interactions have been the defining features of autism. Hence, the need to understand the nature of these difficulties and to find effective treatments for them has been central to autism research and educational practices [5]. Unlike neuro-typical children who learn how to be social and interactive by watching how others talk, play and relate to each other, enjoy the give-and-take of social engagement and initiate, maintain and respond to interactions with others, children with autism often do not show the expected development of early social interaction skills. They are often socially avoidant, socially indifferent and awkward. Autistic children avoid social contact by having a tantrum or running away from people who attempt to interact with them. They seek social contact with people only when they want something. Factors that may affect development of social behavior are described below.

- Theory of Mind: Many children with autism also show profound empathy deficits. They develop a limited appreciation or no appreciation at all, of other people's feelings and ideas. They don't recognize and respond to faces as do normal children, and they thus do not learn that each face belongs to an individual separate person. To the severely autistic child, his/her own feelings and ideas are the only feelings and ideas that appear to exist. Autistic children may have no reaction to another person's crying, for example. They may have no idea that their words and actions affect other people. Many autistic children are completely unaware of their surroundings and other people in their surroundings. It is impossible for some autistic children to take another person's perspective without deliberate training. For individuals with autism, it does not come naturally to consider other people's perspective. This makes it difficult for them to understand how others think and feel [6]. Clinicians and researchers call this inability to consider other's perspective as deficit in *theory of mind*. Theory of mind, the ability to attribute mental states to self and others in order to understand and predict behavior, is an area of weakness among individuals in the autism spectrum. The development of theory of mind begins in infancy, as does the shift from the typical course that is seen in children with autism spectrum disorders. While the peak in theory of mind development occurs in typical children from the age of 3 to 4, mental state understanding in individuals within the autism spectrum often continues to be conspicuously absent throughout the lifespan and leads to significant social and communicative challenges.

- Play Behavior: Play is considered a key social behavior. Children play, regardless of age, so this is a behavior that is typically found in the behavioral repertoires of all children. To teach play to children with autism is to teach them skills that other typically developing children have and give them a common ground, a common language to engage with others. Play phases occur in developmental stages that typically developing children go through, so play is not only for fun, but for a purpose. Children learn about social interaction and language through play. As children with autism have trouble in symbol use and joint attention, understanding another's perspective, participating in pretend play and using imitative skills are difficult for many of them. They are more self-centered than selfish. When involved in joint play, there can be a tendency to impose or dictate the activity. Social contact is tolerated as long as other children play their game according to their rules. Children with ASD play in a 'bubble' and can resent other children intruding into their activity. They prefer to be left alone and continue their activity uninterrupted. There is a strong preference to interact with adults who are far more interesting, knowledgeable and more tolerant and accommodating to their lack of social awareness. It is often hard for them to enter into play with other children, maintain that play, and be appropriate. The children do not see themselves as members of a particular group and follow own interest rather than that of other children in the group. In fact, while other children have mastered the rules of simple childhood games, these children may not understand what is expected of them in team sports. They are often not interested in competitive sports or team games. Even understanding basic turn-taking may elude them. Most of them are unable to comprehend how or why one would have a sense of satisfaction in knowing that one's opponents felt inferior.

- Comprehending Emotions: Inability to empathize with people may be misinterpreted as a complete lack of the ability to care for others. It is more often a lack of *understanding of emotions*. The child is either confused by the emotions of others or has difficulty expressing own feelings. The child does not display the anticipated range and depth of facial expression. As interaction continues, one is aware that the child is not recognizing or responding to changes in the other person's facial expression or body language. Hands may be moved to describe graphically what to do with objects or express anger or frustration, but gestures or body language based on an appreciation of another person's thoughts and feelings- e.g. embarrassment, consolation or pride- are conspicuously diminished or absent [7]. Subtle clues may not be recognized by a child with Asperger's Syndrome. The child can then be confused and offended when criticized for not complying with the signals of hidden intention. Not only are there problems with the understanding of the emotional expressions of others, but the child's own expression of emotions are unusual, and tend to lack subtlety and precision. A complete stranger may be given a kiss on the lips, or distress is expressed quite out of proportion to the situation. Sometimes they cannot express their anger appropriately. When they are anxious or stressed, they may not be able to let others know how they are feeling and may react violently or aggressively. Additionally, appropriate social interaction in autism is hampered by a tendency to become fascinated by special interest that dominates the child's time and conversation, and the imposition of routines that must be completed. The interest is a solitary pursuit and not that evinced by age peers. A lack of completion of the activity in a routine can lead to distress and anxiety. Researches indicate that insistence on completing an activity in a particular way may be the child's attempt to find patterns and look for rules and organization within environment [8]. Once a pattern has emerged it must be maintained. Thus, establishment of a routine ensures that there is no opportunity for change. As social situations are inherently dynamic, this adherence to routine and limited interest deeply impacts the child's ability to be socially active in appropriate manner.

3. Early intervention

Early intervention (EI) is a system of services provided to children who are disabled, have delayed development or are at risk of delayed development, from birth until about five years of age. To help children with autism it is essential to focus on the earliest years of development, since this is a critically important time for early learning which powerfully affects the child's future life course.

Early intervention, also known as early childhood education, provides a support system for children with developmental disabilities and their families. Early intervention may start as soon as it is evident that the child has a developmental disability or is at risk of acquiring it. The early intervention services ensure that infants and pre-school children develop the core skills in physical, cognitive, communication, socio-emotional and self help domains. Early intervention (EI) services are coordinated so that they enable child's growth and development and support families during the critical early years. For the family, such services help in overcoming the feelings of isolation, stress and frustration, and reduce the cost of providing for special education, rehabilitation and health care needs of the child. EI services follow a multidisciplinary approach, with a variety of therapists and teachers working in collaboration to improve the child's prognosis in every area of development.

To help children with autism it is essential to focus on the earliest years of development, since this is a critically important time for early learning which powerfully affects the child's future life course. The children are actively engaged in an instructional program three to five times a week, through the year. It involves planned intervention organized around relatively brief periods of time for the very young children so that they may receive sufficient adult attention. Since children with autism find it difficult to work in large groups, the EI services for them should follow a structured program of one-on-one training or training in small groups to help attain individual goals.

EI is the most dynamic and critical period in the treatment of autism for one very simple reason: the younger they are, the more 'elastic' their brains are [9]. Recognizing and diagnosing autism before pre-school age has been uncommon until the last few years. But increasingly autism is being identified very early in development. It has been shown that diagnosis can be valid and reliable at 2 years of age, and signs can be recognizable and predictive of autism even from early in the second year of life. In future it is likely that autism will be diagnosed for most children in the toddler age period [18 - 30 months). Very early therapeutic intervention is likely to improve developmental and adaptive outcomes. Trials of early intervention need to focus on training parents to work with their very young children in the key areas of social responsiveness, attention skills, early communication skills, and interactive play. The findings of a study by Ivar Lovaas [10] on early behavioral intervention of children with autism in 1987 showed a significant gain in IQ and that 49% of children who received EI were mainstreamed in regular classrooms.

The guidelines for best practice in early intervention for children with autism [11] recommend the following:

- Preparation: All children on entering intervention programs should have had a comprehensive, multidisciplinary diagnostic assessment from an interdisciplinary team of experienced clinicians and based on national and internationally agreed criteria. Diagnostic evaluations should include interviews with parents/care givers to review the child's developmental history, family history, previous assessments and interventions; collection of information from all professionals involved in the care of the child; paediatric, psychological, and speech pathology examinations to assess communication, relevant health conditions including motor skills, vision, and hearing, and any associated problems such as intellectual disability and anxiety. Additionally, direct observation of the child is important in the assessment of cognitive, social, and communicative (verbal & nonverbal) domains, fine and gross motor, and adaptive functioning using both standardised tests and informal procedures.
- Timing: Intervention should begin as early as possible in the child's life. Since a child at risk of autism can be screened by 16 months the intervention may start immediately.
- Process: All children should have an Individual Family Service Plan (IFSP), for their education, designed to best fit their and their family's needs and strengths, developed in consultation with parents, and reviewed and revised regularly in light of the child's progress and ongoing needs.
- Intensity: Ideally the intervention should be provided for 20 hours a week for two years, with continuing support into, and through the school age years.
- Content and Focus: The content should be autism specific and include teaching joint attention skills, play, and imitation skills; building communication through Alternative and Augmentative Communication (AAC) techniques such as pictures, symbols and signs; developing social interaction and daily living skills; and management of sensory issues and challenging behaviors.
- Settings: The intervention should be delivered in various settings, individually and with peers. Implementation should happen both at the centre and at home. Including age peers

with no disability enhances the quality but it should be done so that peer interaction is adequately supported.

- Program Design and Methods: A high degree of structure in the program is essential, i.e. well organized, regular and predictable, focused on specific objectives, and consistently managed. A supportive teaching environment with modeling, prompting, praise, shaping, and generalization strategies will maximize learning.
- Challenging Behaviors: A functional approach to modifying challenging behaviors includes positive behavior support that consists of teaching alternative appropriate behavior and communication skills to replace challenging behaviors.
- Personnel: Teachers and therapists should be adequately trained in working with children with autism and have knowledge and skills required for their special needs.
- Family Collaboration: Parents need information about autism and services, especially at key times like first diagnosis and school entry. Programs should include parent involvement, such as provision of support, counseling, and parent education to help the child with play, social, and communication skills development, and with management of challenging and repetitive behaviors
- Research and Evaluation of Program: Evaluation of treatment outcomes should be built into EI programs using systematic assessment of the child's social, cognitive, and adaptive functioning before, during, and at the end of the program. Regular and systematic documentation of program process and outcome helps in evaluation.

Collaboration with family or parents is a component of best EI practices. Parents of children who have autism play an important role; they are critical components of the intervention process, without whom gains are unlikely to be maintained. The involvement of parents in implementing intervention strategies designed to help their autistic children has a history stretching back at least three decades [12]. Parental involvement is an integral part of the success of early intervention programs for children with autism. The collaboration between the parent and the professional working with the child in the program is critical to the effectiveness of programs.

Traditionally, the EI for autism has been premised on the use of applied behavioral methods such as discrete trials. However, at times parents find the structure, organization and protocol of behavioral intervention difficult to implement and maintain. Consequently, the program receives inadequate follow up in the child's home. There is a need for interventions that do not require a rigid structure and ensure parental involvement. Hence, in the recent years, EI practices for autism have seen a shift from behavioral methods to developmental approaches.

4. Developmental approach

In a developmental approach, development of a child with autism is compared with the developmental sequence seen in non-disabled children. Early childhood assessment tools are used to determine the patterns of typical development. The skills that the child demonstrates are indicative of his or developmental level. The intervention goals are set for the skills the child failed or partially accomplished during assessment. A developmental approach to intervention is also referred to as child centered approach in which the adult follows the child's lead. It uses materials and activities that suit the child's level in a given area of development. The materials are provided to the child, and the adult facilitates the child' interaction with them so that the child moves towards achieving the pre-set developmental goal. But it is the child's initiative with the material or activities that serves as guideline for the adult's interaction. For example, if a child picks up a toy, the adult may show what can be done with it by demonstration and prompts. Child's preferences decide what should be selected as material, and the adult plays a supportive role to encourage the child's interaction with the material. Unlike the behavioral methods, developmental approach does not require the child to interact with material or carry out an activity in a pre-specified structured manner. The consequences of such interactive behaviors are reinforcements that occur naturally in child's environment. The reinforcements may be internal, such as, happiness at being able to complete a task successfully.

5. The DIR model and floor time

The Developmental, Individual, Relationship-based (DIR) Model, designed by Stanley Greenspan in 1989, provides a framework to understand the functional emotional development and unique profile of every child, and a guide to create emotionally meaningful learning interactions that promote critical functional emotional developmental capacities. The objectives of the DIR Model are to build healthy foundations for social, emotional, and intellectual capacities rather than focusing on skills and isolated behaviors [13]. The DIR describes six milestones as crucial to a child's development. Parents and professionals involved with the child must comprehend how the milestones affect a child's emotional and intellectual growth. The six milestones, namely, Self regulation and interest, Intimacy, Two-way communication, Complex communication, Emotional ideas, and Emotional thinking, are explained below. Individual difference is the unique biologically-based ways each child takes in, regulates, responds to, and comprehends sensations such as sound, touch, and the planning and sequencing of actions and ideas. While children may be very hyper sensitive to touch and sound, others may be hypo sensitive, and still others seek out these sensations. Relationship is described as the learning relationships with caregivers, educators, therapists, peers, and others who tailor their affect based interactions to the child's individual differences and developmental capacities to enable progress in mastering the essential foundations.

Floor time, is central to the DIR model of early intervention. It enables professionals and parents to assess and implement intervention programs that address the unique developmental needs of children with autism. The major element of this approach entails that (a) professionals do floor time with the child (b) parents observe floor time being done with their child, and (c) parents change their style of relating to the child with regard to a given milestone. Floor time is a systematic way of working with a child with autism to help him or her climb the developmental ladder. Floor time intervention aims at taking the child back to the first milestones that the child may have missed in the process of development. With the help of the therapists and parents the child works towards achieving the milestones. This is done through intensive one to one sessions for which parents share equal responsibility with the therapists. According to the DIR/Floor time framework, due to individual processing differences, children with autism do not master the early developmental milestones that are the foundations of learning. Floor time [14] describes six core developmental stages that children with autism have often missed or not mastered:

- Regulation and interest in the world: Infants try and process what they see, hear, and feel. They respond to pleasant face and soothing voice. They learn to enjoy, understand and, use the pleasant feelings and sensations to calm themselves. This helps them learn to take in and respond appropriately to the world around them. This ultimately develops the ability to self regulate.
- Engagement and relationship: Babies learn to bond with their parents very soon. They recognize the parents' face and voice, and want to touch them or be close to them. They enjoy being cuddled and loved by their parents. This process of bonding also builds a relationship of trust between babies and their parents. This trusting relationship enables the child to become a well-adjusted adult later in his or her life. It also forms a stable base for all future relationships. The baby learns that relationships with people can be joyful.
- Two-way communication: Once relationship with parents is developed, the baby realizes that he or she can have an impact on parents. The baby's smile can produce a smile from the parents. If the baby reaches out to mother, she picks him or her up. The baby learns that adults can understand and respond to its communication intents and feelings. A dyad of communication starts slowly. When the baby looks at the mother and reaches out to her – the mother responds by giving eye contact and a hug. In turn the baby may smile, vocalize or touch the mother. Thus a non-verbal dialogue or a two-way communication process may be completed. The baby soon transfers this new ability to other things in the environment. He bangs a toy, it makes a noise, and if he drops his bottle, it breaks. His actions can have an impact not only on his parents but others too. Hence, two-way communication helps babies to learn about them and about the world.
- Complex communication: The non-verbal two way communication slowly becomes complex in nature. While earlier the baby was initiating or responding to a communication by a simple gesture of reaching out or smiling, now he may run towards the mother, and squeal with pleasure. Anger and displeasure may be expressed by pulling, kicking and grabbing or throwing things. Similarly, hugs and kisses are used to express affection. Since, the baby is ambulatory by now, he may take the parent by hand and show them what he wants. Complex communication ability also aid development of creativity. The toddler adds his own ideas to the games that parents play with him. This leads to the emergence of the child's own personality.
- Emotional ideas: Play is a fertile ground for ideas. Using toys and playthings, a child creates a world where toys play roles. So, a teddy is a friend, a doll is a baby and a shoe box

is a car garage. This idea-filled play provides a strong basis for language development. Besides learning to label things, the child now uses dialogue during play with help of the parents. Eventually, he is able to manipulate the ideas to meet his needs. When hungry, he can ask for food; if he needs help he can call his mother instead of crying. He learns about object permanence - that although not visible to him, object do not disappear. Hence, he can feel secure thinking about his parents even when they are not with him. With this ability to use symbols, the child moves on to a higher level of communication and awareness.

- Emotional thinking: When he reaches this stage, a child is ready to connect various ideas into a logical sequence. While in the previous stage he was able to carry out symbolic activities, such as dressing a doll, and banging a toy car into another to simulate a crash, the child is now able to think emotionally. He may dress up the doll for a car ride. At this stage, the child is able to express a wide range of emotions, and through this learns to recognize self. The child now comprehends concept of space and time at a personal level. For example, the child understands that grandmother's house is different from his own, or that if he grabs another child's toys, his own favorite car may later be taken away by that child. The child, by this time, is fully verbal and can use words to express ideas and feelings.

5.1. Floor time method

A typical floor time session is conducted in a child's naturalistic environment and requires the therapist or parent to sit on the floor and work with the child. The purpose is to help the child achieve the stages of development, by taking him back to the milestones that he may have missed. During a session, the parent or therapist follows the child's lead. This helps in establishing relationship between the child and the adult. It is this relationship that slowly enables the child to develop the basic social, emotional and communication abilities. During a floor time session the child learns to engage with others, initiate actions, make own wishes and desires known and the realization that his actions can elicit responses from others. Floor time creates opportunities for children to have dialogues, which are called circles of communication, first without words and later with them, and eventually to imagine and think. Since floor time sessions are child-centered, the activities are motivating to the child as it is he who has chosen them. Additionally, the selecting the child's natural environment for the session also contributes to calming him and improving his comfort level. A floor time session follows the steps given below.

1. Observation: Before starting a session, the adult observes the child. This requires watching the child while he is in the room, observing what interests him, assessing his level of interaction – is he running around or is he sitting quietly. This observation helps the adult determine the child's current emotional state.

2. Approach: Once the adult understands the child's level of emotional functioning, he or she joins the child in whatever the child is doing. If the child sits and merely twirls a toy, the adult follows this play behavior. However, the adult adds value to it by label-

ing the activity in gestures and words. The adult also uses appropriate facial expression and tone of voice to convey own enjoyment in what the child is doing. Such measures enable the adult to open the circle of communication with the child

3. Child's Lead: During a floor time session, the child is the director or leader of activities. The adult's role is to follow the child. The aim here is to support the child's activities and initiatives, and through this to take him to a higher level of emotional functioning.

4. Expand Ideas: As the sessions progress, the adult builds on the child's play initiatives. Now the adult associates daily experiences with the experiences during the play activities. For example, the adult may say "give teddy a bath, like mommy gives you". This planned expansion and addition to child's activities help in development of emotional ideas.

5. Close Circle of Communication: Once the adult engages the child at a level the child currently enjoys, enters the child's activities, and follows the child's lead, he or she now attempts to move the child from a mutually shared engagement toward more increasingly complex interactions, a process known as "opening and closing circles of communication." In a circle of communication, the adult opens the circle by approaching the child, and the child closes the circle by giving a reaction to the adult's comments and gestures. During session many circles may open and close in quick successions as the adult interacts with the child. The process leads to two-way communication.

6. Research support for floor time

The Floor time approach examines the functional developmental capacities of children in the context of their unique biological profile and their family relationships and interactive patterns. A longitudinal study [15] was conducted to determine if children with ASD could overcome the core deficits in social behavior and become empathetic and reflective with floor time intervention. A follow-up study of 16 children diagnosed with (ASD) revealed that with the DIR/Floor time approach, a subgroup of children with ASD can become empathetic, creative, and reflective, with healthy peer relationships and solid academic skills. This suggests that some children with ASD can master the core deficits and reach levels of development formerly thought unattainable with a family-oriented approach that focuses on the building blocks of relating, communicating, and thinking [16].

In another study undertaken by Greenspan and Weider [15] where the progress of 200 children who had earlier received Floor time sessions, was reviewed showed that majority of the children learned to relate and engage with warmth, trust and intimacy; they were able to interact, read and respond to social signals; a subgroup of children developed the capacity for imaginative play, creative use of language and reflective thinking. This sub group was included in mainstream schools where the children developed meaningful relationships with peers.

Josefi and Ryan [17] conducted a case study on a 6 year old boy with severe autism. Video recordings of 16 sessions of play therapy with the child were analyzed qualitatively and quantitatively. The study concluded that this child was able to enter into a therapeutic relationship and demonstrated attachment behavior towards the therapist. Key areas of improvement were in the child's development of autonomy and pretend play, while ritualistic behaviors showed only mild improvement. Changes were also noted in the boy's behavior at home of increased independence and empathy. One implication of this preliminary research is that non-directive play therapy may enhance and accelerate emotional/social development of children with severe autism.

Children with ASD differ from one another—in the ways they engage, relate, and communicate and in the ways they respond to sensations, and plan and sequence their actions. These differences mean that each child requires an intervention approach tailored to his uniqueness, an intervention that must also consider the home setting. According to Costa and Witten [18] the goals of such a program, regardless of the approach used, must be to strengthen the child's core deficits, namely: building the foundations for relating, communicating and thinking. The DIR/Floor time Model is especially beneficial to children with ASD and other developmental and/or emotional challenges.

Solomon et al [19] published an evaluation of The PLAY Project Home Consultation, a widely disseminated program that trains parents of children with autism spectrum disorders in the DIR/Floor time model. Sixty- eight children, 2 to 6 years old (average 3.7 years) completed an 8–12 month program where parents were encouraged to deliver 15 hours per week of 1:1 interaction. Pre/post ratings of videotapes by blind raters using the Functional Emotional Assessment Scale (FEAS) showed significant increases in child subscale scores. That is, 45.5 percent of children made good to very good functional developmental progress. Overall parents' satisfaction with program was 90 percent.

7. Method

The study was experimental in nature and employed a pre-test post-test control group experimental design. It was conducted on children with ASD residing in Mumbai, India. The objectives were to determine the efficacy of floor time approach for developing social behavior in pre-school children with ASD, and to compare the levels of social skill achievement by children who received floor time intervention with those who did not.

7.1. Subjects

Children with ASD within the age group of 3 to 6 years were randomly selected from five pre-schools and intervention clinics located across the city and suburban areas of Mumbai. A total of 26 children participated in the experiment. After selection the children were randomly assigned to treatment and control groups so that both groups had 13 children each.

7.2. Instruments

The Behavioral Scale for Social Skills (BSFS) and Floor time intervention were the primary instruments used in the study. They were developed for the purpose of the research. A brief description of both is given below.

- Behavioural Scale for Social Skills: The BSFS was used as a measure at both pre and post tests. The instrument measured social behaviour under 4 domains –

a. Turn taking: This is one of the bases for development of social skills and inferring others' intentions correctly [20]. Turn taking includes use of play material with an adult and with peers.

b. Two-way communication: As a child enjoys intimacy in a safe and calm manner, he realizes he can have an impact on others. The child expresses a feeling or intention, and his partner responds. This is the beginning of communication. Two-way communication enables the child to enjoy intimacy and initiate interaction through gestures at first and then with words.

c. Understanding of cause and effect: This is a basis for development of thinking skills. The ability to see the relationship between an event and the factors leading to it helps a child decode the world around him. Understanding of cause and effect relationship improves by providing the child the opportunity to explore the environment.

d. Emotional thinking: According to Greenspan, emotional thinking is the ability to build bridges between ideas to make them reality-based and logical. Ideas are linked together into logical sequences and play, and imagination is also more rational.

The BSFS had a total of 20 items. Each item was measured on a 4-point scale based on the category of response, namely, correct response; response with verbal prompt; response with gestural prompt; and response with physical prompt. Whereas correct responses were scored as 4, responses with physical prompts were scored as 1. The selection of items under each sub head of BSFS was done after detailed discussions with developmental psychologists, pre-school teachers, and many parents. In addition, several observations of pre-school children with and without ASD were also made for selection of items. The instrument was pilot tested on children with ASD belonging to the same age group as the subjects.

- Floor time Intervention: Floor time is a comprehensive program for infants, young children, and families with a variety of developmental challenges including ASD. The program aims at enhancing the functional emotional developmental levels and creating those learning relationships that will help the child move ahead in social skills acquisition. Floor time can be tailored to suit the individual needs of children with ASD. Floor time approach was used for treatment in the study. As stated earlier, Floor time approach helps an infant/young child reach the 6 milestones crucial for development of social behavior, namely, self regulation; intimacy; two way communication; complex communication; emotional ideas,; and emotional thinking. However, in this study, the treatment was directed toward achievement of 4 milestones – Turn taking (a component skill in intimacy), Two way communication, Understanding of cause and effect relationship (an important skill for problem solving that enhances complex communication), and Emotional thinking. Various activities were developed for the purpose of enhancing the target skills. Some of the activities are mentioned below.

a. Turn taking: Here the activities selected were done with the authors and then done with peers. Such activities as building block tower, bead stringing, rolling a ball, and throwing ball in a bucket were used for teaching turn taking skills to children.

b. Two-way communication: Training a child to respond to his name, reach out to a plaything, and respond to non-verbal communication such as gestures, facial expressions etc was undertaken to develop the ability for two way communication.

c. Cause and effect: A series of simple activities were done to explain the relationship between an outcome and its cause. Tapping a spoon on a surface, shaking a bell, pressing a toy to produce sound or movement, squeezing a wet sponge, opening a transparent box to obtain a desirable object within, etc. were undertaken to help the children establish the connection between a cause and its effect.

d. Emotional thinking: Pretend play was primarily used for this purpose. Hence, pretend play such as talking on telephone, dressing or feeding the doll (where the authors would at times play out the doll's emotions in the right tone of voice), and playing a shopkeeper etc. were included. The focus was on recognition of emotions. Thus, flash cards of happy and sad faces were used too during the pretend play so that the child was able to understand what did it mean when the 'doll' was 'crying' or the the shopkeeper was 'happy'.

7.3. Procedure

The intervention started after assessing the children's baseline behavior on BSFS. The 26 children were then randomly assigned to experimental and control groups so that both groups had 13 children each. As per the recommended floor time protocol, the researchers observed each child in the experimental group to determine his or her current emotional level, before the commencement of intervention. Each child in the experimental group received 20 sessions of floor time intervention. Each session was of 30 minutes duration. Each session included at least one activity relevant to the pre selected social skills. The sessions started by getting the child's attention by showing a desired object. The researchers used word and simple phrases to describe each activity. The activities were done as given below, and parents were encouraged to observe the sessions.

- Building a block tower began by demonstrating how to make a tower from the four blocks provided on the floor. The child was then asked to lay a block over the one put by the adult. Subsequently, the adult would put another block over it. The adult would then prompt the child to take his or her turn to put a block on top. The activity was repeated with a peer. Now the peer would take the adult's role. The adult would call out each child's name and say ' your turn now ', as they put one block over the other to make a block tower.

- A number of colorful beads were placed on the floor along with a string for the bead stringing activity. The task was first demonstrated, and then used to encourage the child to take turn with an adult and later with a peer in slipping a bead through the string.
- The ' ball rolling ' activity was done by rolling the ball to a child and asking him or her o roll it back to the adult. In case of 5 or 6 year old children, a slight variation was made. The activity was introduced with a peer. Both the child and peer were asked to take turns in throwing the ball to the adult and to each other.
- Throwing the ball in the bucket required that the child identify the bucket first. Subsequently, the task was demonstrated before the child taking turn with the adult and with peer to throw a ball in the bucket.
- Cause and effect activities such as ringing a bell (to produce sound), squeezing a sponge (for water to drip), and opening a box (to get what is inside) were demonstrated and subsequently, taught with prompts and cues. Some fun activities such as blowing soap bubbles were also included as soap bubbles excited the children.
- Calling out the child's name, seeking his attention by showing a preferred object or toy helped in initiating two-way communication. Preferred activities served a dual purpose. They could get the child's attention, but they were also helpful in teaching the child a way to communicate. The adult would have a picture of the preferred activity or toy. The child would be asked to point or pick up the picture in order to get the activity. The adult also used facial expression cards to help the child understand what each expression meant.
- Pretend play was a strong medium for teaching emotional thinking. Pretend play was encouraged using a variety of toys such as dolls, telephone, car, kitchen set, and doctor set etc. The adult would pretend to call the child, and ask the child to pick up the phone and say something. While the child was holding the doll, the adult would prompt him or her to hug and kiss the doll. If the child put the doll away, the adult would convey in appropriate tone and affect how sad the doll was feeling. The child would then be prompted to hold the doll again.
- Taking the lead from the child, the adult would stand at the window if the child was standing there. The adult would then softly describe what they could both see.
- Though all activities were pre-planned, the adult would at times digress to include activities that suited the need of the child on a given day.

While the experimental group children received floor time intervention, the children in the control group received the usual early intervention sessions provided in their educational settings. Post intervention, BSFS was administered again.

Figures 1 to 7 illustrate some of the floor time activities done with the children.

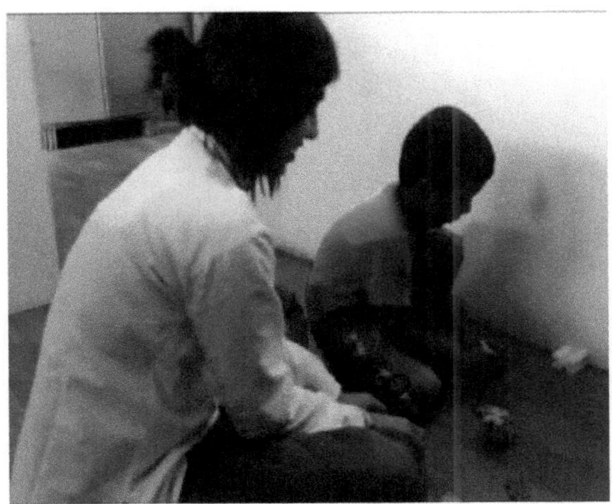

Figure 1. Block tower activity

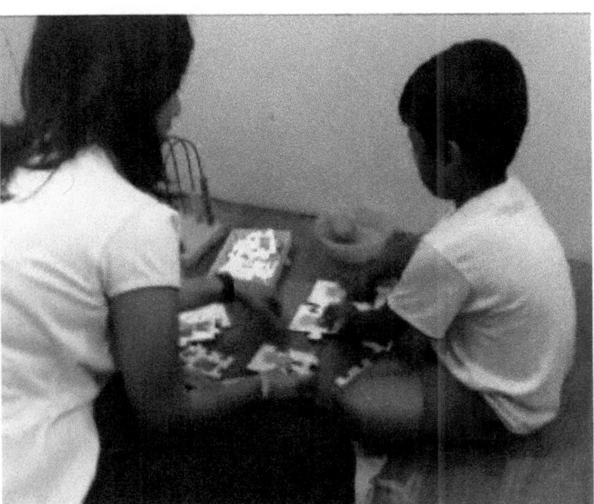

Figure 2. Picture matching

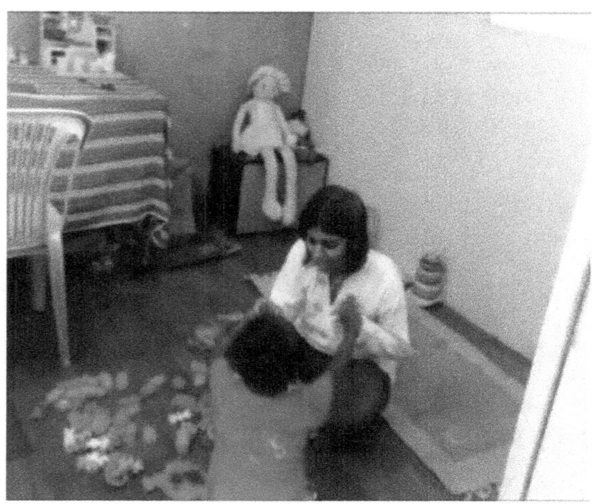

Figure 3. Getting a child's attention

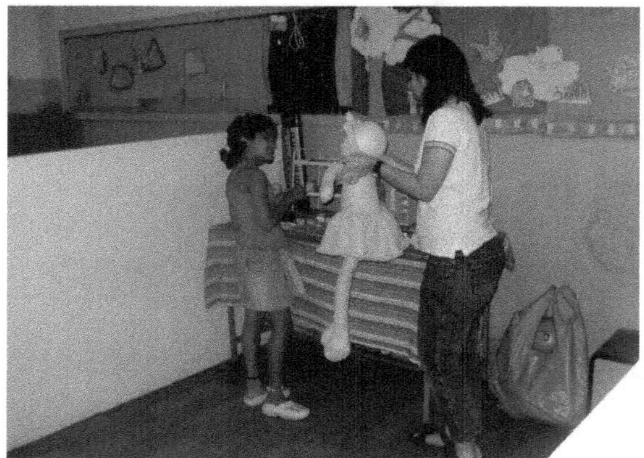

Figure 4. Pretend play with doll

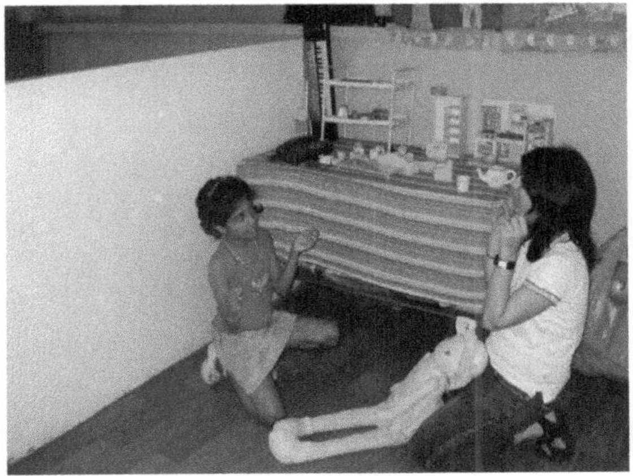

Figure 5. Teaching facial expression

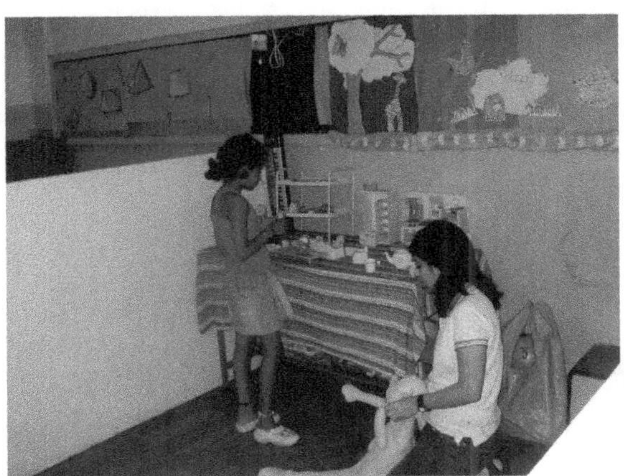

Figure 6. Choice of play things

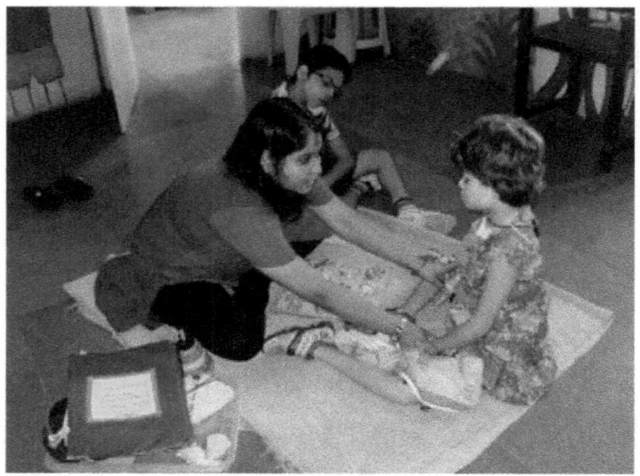

Figure 7. Activity with peer

8. Results

The study was conducted to establish the efficacy of floor time for development of social behavior in pre-school children with ASD. The children who received intervention showed a qualitative change in their interactive behavior. A comparison of their composite mean score on BSFS at baseline with that at post intervention showed a significant difference. The data was analyzed using t-test, as the selection of children was random. Table 1 presents the details.

	Mean	N	df	t-value	Significance
Pre test	34.92	13	12	9.56	p< .0001
Post test	48.38	13			

Table 1. Comparison of Composite Mean Scores on BSFS at Pre and Post Tests

The statistical analysis of data indicated the overall effectiveness of floor time. The average score on BSFS at baseline [34.92] increased post intervention [48.38]. This increase was significant as evident from the obtained t-value [9.56, p<.0001]. That the intervention was effective for all children in the group may be seen from Figure 8 which shows the performance of each child at pre and post intervention conditions

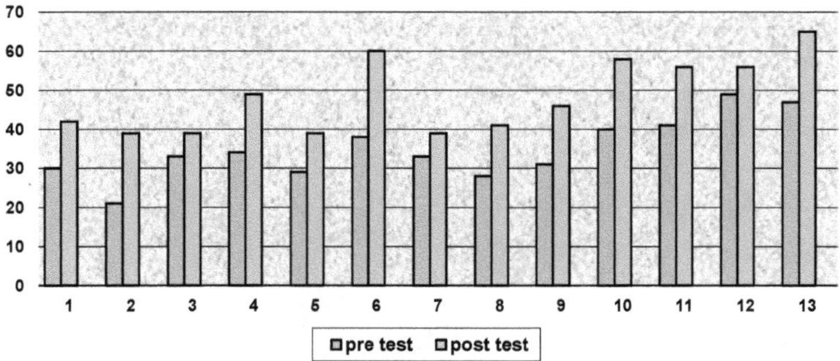

Figure 8. Comparison of individual performance on BSFS

From Figure 8 it is evident that floor time intervention enhanced the social behavior of children, though some gained more from the treatment than others. This variance may be due to initial intra group differences in the children's functioning levels.

Children's scores on selected components of BSFS of turn taking, two way communication, cause and effect and emotional thinking were analyzed individually. On Turn taking skill, the baseline mean [12,38] was significantly lower than the mean score [17.69] post intervention. The derived t-value [5.02] was statistically significant (p<.0002]. An illustration of each child's performance on turn taking skill is provided by Figure 9.

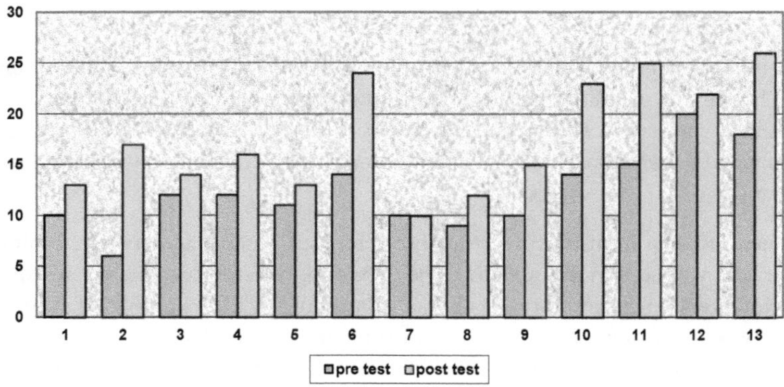

Figure 9. Comparison of individual performance on turn taking

It is evident from Figure 9 that the treatment was effective for all children in the experimental group. All of them gained significantly, except child no. 7 who showed a marginal improvement only. The children's ability to understand the relationship between cause and its effect also improved. Their mean performance on this sub skill post intervention [13.30] was higher than the baseline [8.61]. The derived t-value was significant [7.17, p<.0001]. Each child's performance on cause and effect is depicted in figure 10. The data indicates the effectiveness of floor time as a method to develop the understanding of cause and effect relationship in children with ASD.

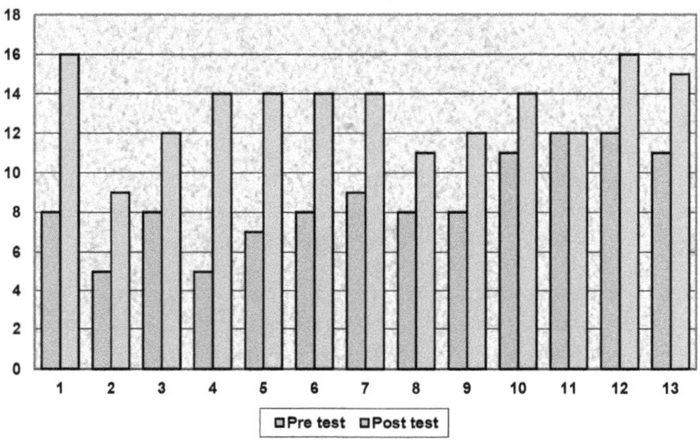

Figure 10. comparioson of individual performance on cause and effect relationship

When performances on two-way communication skills were compared, a similar trend was evident. The mean score at baseline [6.31] was lower than that post intervention [8.69] and the difference was statistically significant (t=5.72, p<.0001]. Individually too, children improved as may be seen from figure 11. All children gained on the ability for two-way communication.

Lastly, when the data from BSFS were analyzed for performance on emotional thinking, a significant gain was seen in this area too. The difference between baseline mean score [7.38] and post intervention mean score [8.84] was significant (t-value=3.5, p<.004]. Though this difference was significant when means were compared, individually all children did not gain from the intervention. Whereas most children showed an enhancement in emotional thinking from pre to post intervention, performance of some remained the same as what it was at baseline. Figure 12 presents the data on emotional thinking. Since, emotional thinking is the last and the most complex of the six milestones; it is possible that these children required more time to achieve this skill than what was given during the 20 sessions of intervention. However, these children improved their performance on the earlier sub-skills of turn taking, two-way communication and understanding of cause and effect relationship.

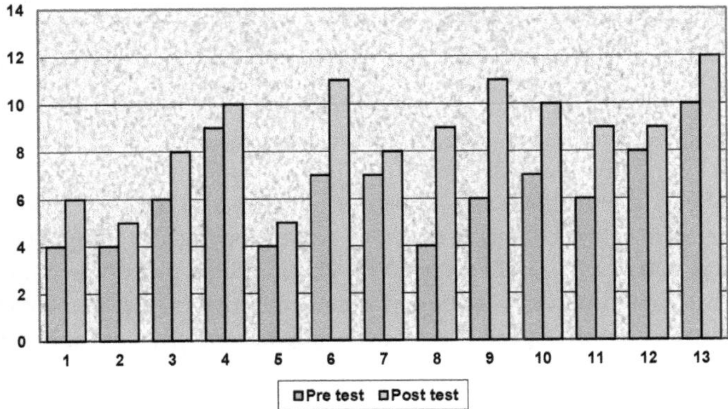

Figure 11. Comparison of individual performance on two-way communication

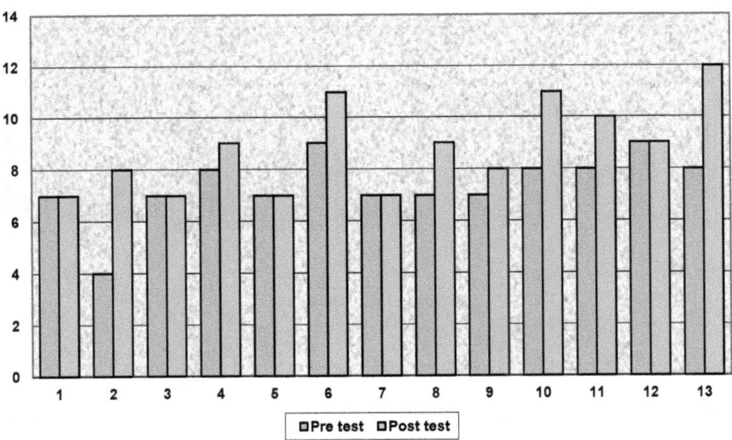

Figure 12. Comparison of individual performance on emotional thinking

The second objective of the study was to compare the performance of children in the experimental group with that of those in control group. As mentioned earlier, the participant children were randomly selected from 5 pre-schools and intervention clinics. Hence, when the study commenced all children were on some kind of early intervention program. The study, in effect, determined the efficacy of floor time in comparison with other early intervention strategies. In order to do this, the post intervention performance on BSFS by both groups was analyzed. The mean score of experimental group was compared with that of control group. The data analysis is presented in Table 2.

	Mean	N	df	t-value	Significance
Experimental	48.38	13	24	3.08	p<.0.005
Control	37.46	13			

Table 2. Comparison of Post test performance of experimental and control groups

Comparison of post intervention mean scores of experimental and control groups showed a significant difference between the two, in favour of the experimental group. The resultant t-value [3.08] was statistically significant (p<.005]. This indicated that in comparison to other measures for early intervention, floor time was more effective in development of social behavior of children with ASD. Figure 13 provides a graphic representation of this difference

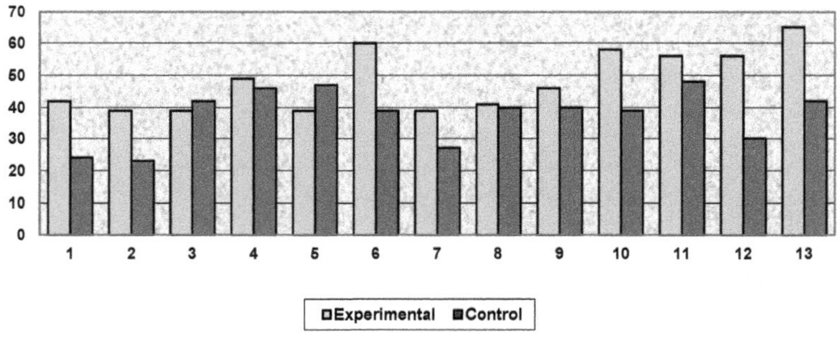

Figure 13. Comparison of post intervention performance of experimental and control groups

It is evident from Figure 13 that except for child no. 3 and child no. 5, all children in experiment group achieved higher scores on BSFS than the control group children. Most children's scored significantly higher than their control group peers. A comparative analysis of both group's mean performance on each sub skill i.e. turn taking (TT), two-way communication (TWC), cause and effect (C&E), and emotional thinking (ET), within BSFS is presented in Figure 14.

The children who received floor time intervention performed better on an average than those who were in the control group. However, the performance gap between the two groups was not uniform across all sub skills. On emotional thinking skill, the average performance of both groups was nearly same with control group's mean less than 2 points below that of experimental group.

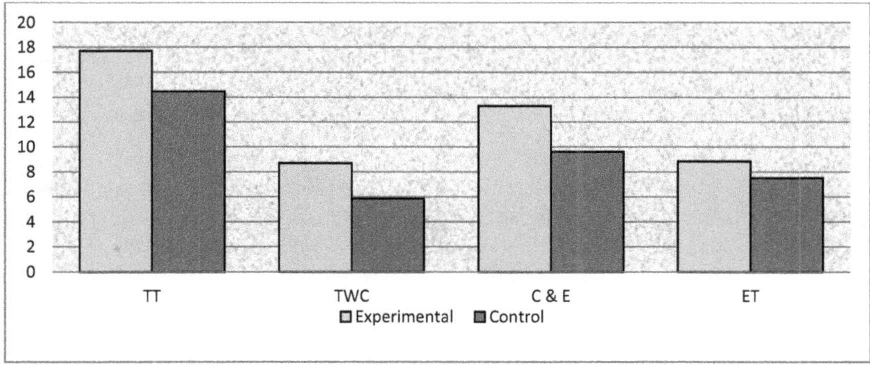

Figure 14. Comparison of experimental and control group on sub skills of BSFS

9. Discussion

Unlike neuro-typical children who learn how to be social and interactive by watching how others talk, play and relate to each other, enjoy the give-and-take of social engagement and initiate, maintain and respond to interactions with others, children with autism often do not show the expected development of early social interaction skills. Promoting the social development of infants and toddlers with ASD is one of the primary goals of early intervention services, as is facilitating the ability of young children with social delays to develop appropriate friendships. With early and intensive intervention, the seemingly pervasive social skill deficits of many children with ASD can be remediated[21]. To successfully target these important skills, intervention efforts, even within early intervention, should include: (a) regular access to typical peers, (b) thoughtful planning of meaningful social situations embedded throughout the day, (c) the use of "social" toys, (d) multiple-setting opportunities (home inclusive, community-based) to practice emerging social skills, and (e) intensive data collection in order to make midcourse corrections to existing intervention plans [22]. Poor social skills are an impediment to child's success in classroom, and can also be the cause of behavioral problem. Accordingly, teaching social skills is a common educational objective for children who have autism [23]. However, while teaching variables such as age, developmental and functional levels and sensory profile of each should be considered. Floor time which is based on the developmental approach takes care of the child's developmental level and emphasizes building the milestones that the child may have missed during his or her period of growth. Rather than focusing on teaching a child to speak a few words to interact, Greenspan suggests that the child's gestural system should be worked upon first for language to flow in naturally rather than by rote, thus focusing on the developmental ladder. As the child climbs the developmental ladder he or she becomes more and more regulated and forms a sense of self. In the study the authors chose age and functionally appropriate activities for helping a child achieve the given milestones for social behavior. The individual sessions during which the adult followed the child's lead, prompted and encouraged the child effort to participate, and provided the opportunity to practice the skill with a peer contributed to the significant increase in each child's performance from pre to post intervention on BSFS.

According to the Colorado guidelines [24] early intervention strategies must involve building of positive relationships between adults (parents and caregivers) and the infant or toddler. The intent should be to teach the child that parents and caregivers can be relied on as stable, secure, and safe figures that provide nurturance, comfort, pleasure and guidance. Developing attachments is a challenge for a young child with ASD, so special efforts are required, even when signs of a child's interest are not apparent. This might require that a parent or caregiver identify the activities, objects, settings, and interactions that the child finds pleasurable and provide those events and items to the child contingent on a social interaction behavior (rather than non-contingently in a manner meant to keep a child satisfied without social interaction). A tickle game might be initiated with a child and then interrupted by the caregiver with the expectation that the child look at the adult or repeat a gesture to continue. A key objective of efforts to form positive relationships is to ensure that the interactions are pleasurable and that they are associated with the child receiving input that is consistent with needs and interests. Importantly, successful efforts to form strong, positive bonds when a child is very young result in a subsequent relationship in which an adult has considerable influence over a child's behavior and this influence can be essential for the guidance and instruction that the adult (parent or other caregiver) must provide on an ongoing basis. The floor time intervention addressed the issues mentioned above. Activities selected were simple and manageable for the children. Most activities were demonstrated before the child was required to participate. For children with autism, visually organized tasks are easier to learn [25]. During intervention the adult often provided model/picture of a task to be done e.g. block tower, completed puzzle, picture and symbol cards etc. Intervention sessions were built around child's motivation and interests. Most early intervention programs for children with ASD are based on behavioral approach and use discrete trial training. Though evaluations have shown acquisition of learning and behavioral development in several children [26], behavioral approach does not suit all children and families. Strict protocol of timing, intensity, structure, and quality of therapist training influences the success of behavioral interventions. In contrast, floor time encourages naturalistic interactions to develop the core skills. It takes into account the inherent bonding and affection parents have for the child, and guides the parent to modify and channelize their interactions to suit the developmental level of the child. As stated earlier, the children selected for the study attended pre-school and intervention clinics. Thus control group children also received early intervention while floor time intervention was given to the experimental group. However, the experimental group children performed better on selected social skills at the end of the intervention period. The significantly higher achievement of social skills by experimental group children may be attributed to the child-centric naturalistic interactions that occurred during the floor time intervention.

10. Conclusion

Early intervention is very important for enhancing the development of infants and toddlers with disabilities, and they are especially crucial in determining the future language, social and behavioral outcomes of very young children with ASD [27]. A primary consideration of programs for young children with ASD is to provide an environment that is designed to prevent problem behaviors, promote engagement and participation, and facilitate successful interactions with typically developing peers. Getting the child to engage with materials and activities may prevent challenging behavior occurrence and promote appropriate social behavior [28]. Results of this research support the above findings. Floor time principles state that development begins with a shared world between the caregiver and the young child. The goal is to help the child with ASD emerge from its own world and enter this shared world in order to develop his or her functional and emotional capacities. Floor time achieves this by encouraging child to engage in age and level appropriate play activities with adults and later with peers. The outcomes indicate the effectiveness of Floor time as a method for early intervention of children with autism. The findings of the study may be useful for families who are in need of evidence based and suitable early intervention for children with ASD.

Acknowledgements

The authors wish to thank the children who participated in this study, and are grateful to the children's parents, teachers, therapists, and administrators of the schools and intervention clinics for their support.

Author details

Rubina Lal and Rakhee Chhabria

Department of Special Education, SNDT Women's University, Mumbai, India

References

[1] Autism Society of America (2006). *Defining Autism.* Available from http://www.autismsociety.org (accessed May. 8, 2012)

[2] American Psychiatric Association (2000). Diagnostic and Statistical Manual of Mental Disorders (4th ed. TR). Washington DC

[3] Young, R. Brewer, N. Pattison, C. (2003). Parental identification of early behavioralabnormalities in children with autistic disorder. Autism, 7, 125-143.

[4] Volkmar, F. Chawarska, K. Klin, A. (2005). Autism in infancy and early childhood. Annual Review of Psychology, 56, 315-36.

[5] Lal, R. and Ganesan, K. (2011) Children with Autism Spectrum Disorders:Social Stories and Self Management of Behaviour British Journal of Educational Research1(1): 36-48, 2011SCIENCEDOMAIN international

[6] Richard, G. J. (2000). The source for treatment methodologies in autism. East Moline, IL: Lingui Systems

[7] Attwood, T. (1988). Asperger's syndrome: A guide for parents and professionals. London. Jessica Kinsley.

[8] Baron-Cohen, S. (2003a). The essential difference: The truth about the male and female brain. New York: Basic Books

[9] Martin, N. (2009) Art as an early intervention tool for children with autism. Jessica Kinsley Publishers, PA.USA

[10] Lovaas OI. Behavioral treatment and normal educational and intellectual functioning in youngautistic children. J Consult Clin Psychol. 1987;55(1):3–9

[11] Prior,M & Robert, J. (2006) Early Intervention for Children with Autism Spectrum Disorders: for Best Practices http://www.health.gov.au/internet/main/publishing.nsf/content/D9F44B55D7698467CA257280007A98BD/$File/autbro.pdf (accessed June 20, 2012)

[12] Diggle, T.T.J, and McConachie, H.H.R. (2009) Parent-mediated early intervention for young children with autism spectrum disorder (Review) http://onlinelibrary.wiley.com/doi/10.1002/14651858.CD003496/pdf/standard (accessed on August, 2012)

[13] http://www.icdl.com/DIRFloortime.shtml (accessed on Sept. 1, 2012)

[14] Greenspan, S.I., and Wieder, S. (1998). The child with special needs. Encouraging intellectual and emotional growth. Perseus Publishing, Massachusetts

[15] Wieder, S. and Greenspan, S.I., (2005). Can children with autism master the core deficits and become empathetic,creative, and reflective?:A Ten to Fifteen Year Follow-Up of a Subgroup of Children with Autism Spectrum Disorders (ASD) Who Received a Comprehensive Developmental, Individual-Difference, Relationship-Based (DIR)Approach. Journal of Developmental and Learning Disorders Vol 9: 39-60

[16] Greenspan, S.I., and Wieder, S. (1997b). developmental patters and outcomes in infants and children with disorders in relating and communicating: A chart review of 200 children with autistic spectrum diagnoses. Journal of Developmental and Learning Disorders. 1: 87-141

[17] Josefi, O.,Ryan, V (2004). Non-directive play therapy for young children with autism: A case study Children. Clinical Child Psychology & Psychiatry. Vol 9 (4), 533-51.

[18] Costa G & Witten MR(2009). Pervasive Developmental Disorders. In Mowder, Rubinson & Yasik (Eds), Evidence-Based Practice in Infant and Early Childhood Psychology. Wiley.

[19] Solomon, R., J. Necheles, C. Ferch, and D. Bruckman (2007) Pilot study of a parent training program for young children with autism: The P.L.A.Y. Project Home Consultation program. Autism 11, no. 3 205-224.

[20] Nadel, J.: Early imitation and a sense of agency. In: Proceedings of the 4th international workshop on epigenetic robots (2004) http://tivipe.com/TVPresearch/62430115.pdf (accessed on Sept.19, 2012)

[21] McGee, G., Daly, T. & Jacobs, H.A. (1993). Walden preschool. In S. L. Harris & J.S. Handleman (Eds.), Preschooleducation programs for children with autism. Austin, TX:Pro-Ed.

[22] Strain, P. S., & Danko, C. D. (1995). Caregivers' encouragement of positive interaction between preschoolers with autism and their siblings. Journal of Emotional and Behavioral Disorders, 3, 2–12.

[23] Weiss, M.J., & Harris, S.L. (2001). Teaching social skills to people with autism. Journal of Behavior Modification. 25, 785-802

[24] Early Intervention Colorado Autism Guidelines for Infants and Toddlers (2010). Developed by the Universityof Colorado Denver, PELE Center, under contract with the Colorado Department of Human Services, Division for Developmental Disabilities. www.eicolorado.org (accessed on July 2,2012)

[25] Lal, R. and Shahane, A. (2011). TEACCH Intervention for autism. In T.Williams (Ed.) Autism Spectrum Disorders-From Genes to Environment. In Tech, Croatia

[26] Lal, R and Lobo, S. (2007). Discrete trial training and development of pre learning skills in intellectually impaired children with autism. Journal of Rehabilitation Council of India. 3, 1&2: 15-23

[27] National Resource Council, (2002). Educating Children with Autism. National Academic Press, Washington

[28] Strain, P., & Schwartz, I. (2009). Positive behavior support and early intervention for young children with autism: Case studies on the efficacy of proactive treatment of problem behavior. In W. Sailor, G. Dunlap, G. Sugai, & R.H. Horner (Eds). Handbook of positive behavior support (pp. 107–123). New York

Chapter 7

Early Communication Intervention for Children with Autism Spectrum Disorders

Gunilla Thunberg

Additional information is available at the end of the chapter

1. Introduction

The main purpose of this chapter is to present the results of a review of communication interventions for children aged 0-6 years with autism spectrum disorders and to formulate recommendations for an evidence-based practice. The study, including 20 reviews and 27 primary studies, specifically focus interventions targeting children with diagnosis within the autism spectrum being on an early communicative level.

2. Communication in children with Autism Spectrum Disorders (ASD)

2.1. Difficulties with communication and language as part of the spectrum

Major advances have been made over the two past decades in understanding the social-communication difficulties of children with ASD, resulting in greater emphasis on early social-communication features in the diagnostic criteria. Most parents of children with autism first begin to be concerned that something is not quite right in their child's development because of early delays or regressions in the development of speech [1]. Problems with communication, in terms of both understanding and expression, are often said to be one of the main causes of the severe behaviour problems that are common among persons with severe autism and mental retardation [2]. The lack of meaningful, spontaneous speech by age five has been associated with poor adult outcomes [3,4,5,6]. Certainly, communication and communication problems are at the heart of what ASD is all about.

Although all persons diagnosed with autism have problems with communication, their type and degree vary a lot and the work of identifying different subgroups has just begun. It has been estimated that between one-third [7] and one-half [8] of children and adults with autism have no speech. However, more recent research results indicate that the proportion of non-speaking children with ASD is much smaller, approximately 14% to 20%, among those who received very early intervention [9].

Two phenotypes of speaking children with ASD were identified by Tager-Flusberg and Joseph [10]: children with normal linguistic abilities (phonological skills, vocabulary, syntax, and morphology) and children with impaired language that is similar to the phenotype found in specific language impairment. Another potential subgroup may experience verbal dyspraxia or dyspraxia of speech [11; 12; 13]. Voluntary motor control is disturbed in children with dyspraxia, which also affects their ability to imitate. The new research on the role of the 'mirror neurons' in the parietal and frontal lobes may provide some answers on the relationships between motor control and imitation but also on the possible link with the development of intersubjectivity [11].

In spite of the heterogeneity of language abilities in children with ASD, social-communication or pragmatic impairments are universal across all ages and ability levels [14]. According to Wetherby [15], the social-communication deficits in children with ASD can be organized into two major areas: (1) the capacity for joint attention and (2) the capacity for symbol use. Since joint attention emerges before words, this deficit may be more fundamental and a number of longitudinal studies provide evidence of a relationship between joint attention and language outcomes [16, 17]. According to Wetherby [15] p. 11, 'deficits in initiating and responding to joint attention have a cascading effect on language development since language learning occurs within the context of the modelling by the caregiver of words that refer to objects and words that are jointly regarded'. Wetherby [15] states that deficits in imitation and observational learning are other main causes of the problems with symbol use experienced by children with ASD. Learning shared meanings, imitating and using conventional behaviours, and being able to decontextualize meaning from the context constitute the symbolic deficits in children with ASD [13].

2.2. Development of communication and language in children with ASD

Because autism is usually not diagnosed until age three or four, there is relatively little information about language in very young children with autism [10]. Retrospective studies using parent reports and/or videotapes collected during infancy, together with studies of children considered likely to develop autism, show severely delayed language acquisition with respect to both receptive and expressive skills [18, 19, 20]. Another typical phenomenon described by 25% of parents of children with ASD is language loss after initially developing some words [21]. Lord, Schulman, and DiLavore [22] found that this language regression is unique to autism and does not occur in other children with developmental delays. Chawarska et al. [21] hypothesize that these early-acquired speech-like productions are lost by children with ASD because the link between these expressions and a network of symbolic communication fails. There is significant variability in the rate at which language progresses among children with ASD who do acquire speech.

The few longitudinal studies of language acquisition in children with ASD suggest that progress within each domain of language follows similar pathways as it does in typically developing children [9, 12]. However, the speech of children with ASD is also characterized by some typical deviations. One of the most salient aspects is the occurrence of echolalia, which can be either immediate or delayed. Although some echolalia seems to be self-stimulating, both types of echolalia can serve communicative purposes for the speaker [12]. At an early stage of language development, this may be the only way in which the child can actually produce speech. Tager-Flusberg et al. (1990) found that, over the course of development, echolalia rapidly declined for all the children with ASD and Down's syndrome in their study. Another prominent feature of language in children with ASD is general problems with deixis, which are most often manifested as pronoun confusion [10]. Features such as vocal quality, intonation and stress patterns often result in problems for persons with ASD, although there is a lack of research in this field. Taken together, the findings suggest that the difficulties are due not only to problems in social intent but also to problems affecting a more basic aspect of vocalization [12].

Less research attention has focused on the comprehension skills of individuals with ASD although deviations in response to language and comprehension have been found to be strong indicators of ASD [18]. According to Tager-Flusberg et al. [14], it seems that ASD children 'not only may have limited ability to integrate linguistic input with real-world knowledge but also may lack knowledge about social events used by normally developing children to buttress emerging language skills and to acquire increasingly advanced linguistic structures' [12, p. 350].

The pragmatic aspects of language have been studied in numerous ways. Children with autism share important similarities across different language levels [12]. The speech acts that are missing or rarely used in the conversations of children with autism often concern social, rather than regulatory, uses of language [22]. Ramberg, Ehlers, Nydén, Johansson, and Gillberg [24] found that children with ASD were impaired in taking turns during dyadic conversations. A higher proportion of initiations rather than responses was found in a study [25]. Although the basic intention to communicate often exists, the person with autism has impaired skill in participating in communicative activities involving joint reference or shared topics [12, p. 354].

3. Interventions to support communication and language development in children with ASD

3.1. History and different theoretical approaches

The first reports on language interventions were published in the mid-1960s. The intervention at that time built on the operant tradition developed by Skinner during the 1950s. The teaching sessions in this method, referred to as discrete trial teaching or didactic teaching, are marked by a high level of adult control and direction, massed-practice periods for preselected tasks, and precise antecedent, teaching, and reinforcement practices. The learner is in a responder role, and the teacher has a directive role [11]. The strength of the didactic behavioural approach is primarily that it has demonstrated efficacy in many studies, using a variety of treatment settings and treatment deliverers, with both single-subject and group designs [11]. Limitations on this approach as a language-training method were recognized early on, with the children's lack of generalization being a core problem [26].

The pragmatic understanding of communication was fully developed after the operant teaching methods were first developed [11]. The current scientific understanding of communication and language development stems from the 1970s and 1980s, when it was demonstrated that language develops from the preverbal social exchanges of infants with important others (Bates, 1976). According to Rogers [11 p. 149], 'current research, building primarily on the work of Wetherby [13, 15, 23], Prizant [13], and Mundy, Sigman and Kasari [17], has demonstrated that young children with autism lacked these early building blocks of communication, involving social initiative, joint attention, social and emotional reciprocity, and the use of gestures to co-ordinate social exchanges.

In 1968, an important study was published by Hart and Risley [27]. Very positive results were obtained with an intervention in which the principles of operant teaching were applied in the child's natural environment. The term 'incidental teaching' was used for this approach, in which the natural environment is deliberately structured to highlight the function of the targeted language form. This intervention produced much better results with respect to maintenance and generalization and stimulated development and research in the field [11]. According to Rogers [11, p. 153], the effectiveness of this approach results from four factors: (1) child language functions to achieve child-chosen goals and child-chosen reinforcers, which strengthen their power; (2) the focus is on child communication skills that are functional in all settings; (3) the social functions of language are highlighted; (4) emphasis on child motivation and natural reinforcers adds a positive element to the interactions, which may enhance memory for learning.

The third major approach in the field of communication intervention for children with ASD is the developmental pragmatic approach. The most elaborated programme for treatment, the SCERTS (Social-Communication, Emotional Regulation, Transactional Support) model [28] focuses on functional communication. This approach bears many resemblances to the behavioural naturalistic teaching methods. More emphasis is, however, placed on developing nonverbal behaviours prior to verbal communication and on the use of Augmentative and Alternative Communication (AAC) systems to assist in the development of verbal communication [11]. Today many models combine behavioural techniques and social-interactionist approaches, such as Enhanced Milieu Teaching, developed by Kaiser and colleagues [29], The Denver Early Start [30], Caregiver Mediated Joint Engagement Intervention for Toddlers with Autism [31], Focus parent training for toddlers with autism [32]. The strength of the developmental model is its strong basis in the science of communication development. Its weaknesses include the lack of treatment manuals and the fact that it requires considerable knowledge on the part of the therapist [11].

3.2. Early communication intervention

3.2.1. Why early communication intervention?

Several new research findings point to the importance of an early start of communication intervention. The most essential of these are:

- Difficulties in understanding and expressing communication is very closely linked to the development of challenging behaviors in individuals with autism [2].
- Communication and language are pivotal for the development of several other cognitive constructs or competencies, such as:
  - Reading and writing.
  - Theory of Mind [33].
- Communication ability predicts outcome with respect to functioning and quality of life in adults with autism spectrum disorders [3].
- The severity of communication difficulties in preschool-aged children is correlated to the perceived level of stress in their parents [34].
- Communication is one of the most important factors for the participation in daily activities of young disabled children [35].
- According to several guidelines, among these NRC (National Research Council) in the United States, functional communication and social interaction should be prioritized in early intervention programs given to children with ASD.

Furthermore, interactional research done on children with communicative impairments and their parents has shown that the responsive communication style that characterizes parents of typically developing children is often replaced by a more directive style in parents of children with communicative impairments. Besides this impact on quality, quantity is also affected, in that the rate of communication occasions in these families tend to decrease. This adds a cumulative negative effect on the communication development due to less stimulation and experience [36]. Research has also shown that children with ASD whose parents used a responsive style during preschool years in general had better communication and languages skills when they were followed up as teen-agers [37].

3.2.2. Early communication intervention methods or programs

There are many intervention programs for children with ASD that focus on communication. Some of these are more specifically aimed at communication whilst others include communication and language as a part of a comprehensive early intervention program. Some programs (indirect interventions) focus on the parent or partner usually by guiding and teaching parents, individually or in groups (courses). Other intervention programs focus more on the training of the child (direct interventions). Today it is common that early intervention programs include both indirect and direct aspects: education and tutoring of parents and training of the child.

Another dimension of great importance in early communication intervention concerns the degree of child focus. To have a child focus means that the motivation of the child and the developmental level is decisive in what is done during intervention. The adult follows the lead of the child and the place for training is where the child is, often the floor. In this way it's not necessary to use reinforcements or rewards since the child is already interested and motivated. To get the child to train and focus the intended skills or functions different behavioural techniques are often used. At the other end of this dimension we find the more traditional didactic training situation where the adult trainer or therapist follows and uses a predefined set of activities and materials during a training session. The specific behavioural techniques; prompts and reinforcements used during the session are often also specified or planned. The child is expected to follow the lead of the adult and it is typical that the training is held the child and the adult sitting face-to-face at a table. It is more typical that child-focused interventions are provided during daily activities in the natural environment of the child; at home and/or in preeschool, whilst didactic training is provided at a clinic, at least during the introduction of new materials and training activities.

Still another difference between programs that might be seen as a dimension is the degree to which augmentative and alternative communication (AAC) is included. In some programs these strategies, in the form of manual signs, symbols and pictures and speech-generating devices (SGDs, today often Apps used on an iPad, smartphone or other platform), are included already from the start to promote communication and build language, whilst in other programs AAC strategies are not included, but instead seen as a last resort when training of speech has failed.

3.2.2.1. Education and tutoring of parents and staff

The most common intervention of this type is parental education. The internationally most wide-spread parental education programs most probably are the courses developed by the Canadian Hanen Centre [38]. The course being developed for children within the autism spectrum is called More Than Words and includes eight group sessions for the parents and three "home-visits" by the Speech-language pathologist. During these visits the interaction between the child and the parent is videotaped and the parents are given feed-back and further guidance how to improve communication and use of the strategies being taught during the course. The Hanen courses is a developmental approach and teaches responsive strategies to the parents adding some behavioural techniques to stimulate communication learning within the frames of child-focused natural interaction in the home [38]. A new parental course called ComAlong has been developed in Sweden and now is spreading in northern Europe [39]. ComAlong include eight group sessions focusing on responsive strategies and environmental teaching but also puts a large focus on the use of augmentative communication strategies in the home setting [39]. The parents are provided with picture boards so they can use aided language modeling in their homes [39, 40].

3.2.2.2. *Comprehensive intervention programs*

Training of communication, language and speech is most often an important part in the different comprehensive programs, addressing different skills and problems, that has been developed for young children within the autism spectrum. Some of these are built on behavioural theories, others on developmental pragmatic approaches. There seems to be a trend that the programs being developed and researched during the last decade, specifically for young children with autism, are more eclectic. The background theories are often described as developmental pragmatic whilst ABA (Applied Behavior Analysis) techniques are used to strengthen the teaching practices. Most often these comprehensive programs include both direct training to the child and indirect intervention parts in that parents and/or staff in the close network of the child are given education, training and/or guidance.

3.2.2.3. *Augmentative and Alternative Communication — AAC*

AAC comprises different methods and modes of communication such as body communication, concrete objects, manual signs, graphic symbols or speech-generating devices. Historically, the first studies describing AAC techniques being used for individuals with autism appeared in the 1970s; they reported on the use of sign language to improve communication [41]. These studies appeared at the same time as the unsatisfactory results of spoken-language-training programmes were being published. Studies by, for example, Lovaas et al. [26] reported little change after many hours of intensive treatment, and the results were particularly poor for the children whose comprehension and vocal skills were most impaired [41]. Initially, most signing programmes were built on formal sign language systems, but it became evident that these were often too complex and abstract, and so specially adapted systems were developed and implemented. Sign-based programmes spread rapidly in schools for children with autism in many countries.

During the 80's and the 90's a gradual change in AAC intervention for persons with autism, was seen, as visual-graphic communication was more in focus. Mirenda and Erickson [42] explain that the shift away from the use of signing to visual-graphic communication occurred as a result of research findings in three main areas: imitation, iconicity, and intelligibility. In addition to the evidence of a generalized imitation deficit in autism, there were also studies showing that some children with ASD had extremely poor sign imitation skills [43] due to difficulties with motor planning, control and execution [44]. According to Howlin [41], the shift from the use of manual signs to visual methods was also due to the fact that visual methods had proven to be effective in enhancing general skill acquisition, mainly within the TEACCH programme (Treatment of Education of Autistic and related Communication-handicapped CHildren; [45]) developed during the 1970s. A variety of symbol systems were also developed, beginning with Blissymbolics and Rebus followed by Pictogram and Picture Communication Symbols. The improvements in computer technology made these symbol sets easily available in the form of practical software packages. The development of digital cameras during the 1990s also increased the possibility of including personal photos in AAC systems, which, according to clinical reports, seemed to increase motivation and facilitate understanding of pictures, particularly for individuals with ASD [46].

There are, however, also reports of problems in teaching symbols to children with ASD, mainly in teaching them to use the pictures spontaneously and for communicative functions other than requesting [41]. It was precisely these problems that led Bondy and Frost [47] to develop the method called Picture Exchange Communication System (PECS). PECS is a systematic approach to communication training specifically developed for children with autism. The elements that make PECS different from other visual-graphic techniques are the use of the concrete hand-to-hand exchange of the picture and also the highly prescriptive user manual with its six levels to follow in sequence.

Historically, the use of speech output technologies with individuals with ASD has not been a matter of course [48]. Computer technology was introduced into educational settings for children with autism late, not only in North America, but also in other countries. Professionals feared that people with ASD would become even more aloof if they were encouraged to sit in front of a computer screen. Concerning speech-generating devices (SGDs), a common view was that they would only stimulate echolalia in children with ASD, and that there would be too much noise in the classroom. By the end of the 1990s, scepticism had decreased. This was probably due to reports of some studies of successful computer-assisted instruction (CAI) carried out. The introduction of "app technology "has meant a revolution to the field of speech-generating devices and the first studies of the effects of apps are now being published.

4. Evidence-Based Practice — EBP

The term evidence-based used as a prefix and a denominator of interventions and methods comes from medicine. The term evidence based means that the choices of interventions and assessments are based on a research literature not simply professional experience or previous practice. Evidence-based practice has been important within the area of early communication intervention. The behavioural intervention tradition with its roots in the research clinic has produced a lot of high-quality research during the years. Other types of interventions has been less researched and sometimes have used methods and produced data that are different so that comparisons of effects are hard or impossible to do. This has also led to an interesting discussion of how to do EPB within the field of communication intervention. Ralph W. Schlosser, professor at NorthEastern University, USA, has been of great importance in this respect. Partly because he is spreading knowledge about evidence-based practise (EBP) and due to the many thorough compilations of research that he has done, but also in demonstrating the problems and shortcomings using EBP in relation to the field of augmentative communication intervention [49]. One of these problems concerns the use of the Randomized Controlled Trial or Study (RCT) as the golden standard, as RCTs are almost non-existent within the AAC field. There are many reasons to this but the main ones are that (1) children with communicative disabilities are so heterogeneous and (2) that randomization is extremely difficult to put through due to ethical reasons.

Schlosser has therefore suggested an alternative evidence hierarchy placing the meta-analysis on top [49, 50]. Schlosser and several other prominent authors within the field of communication intervention research designs recommend the use of well-controlled single-subject research designs that can form the base for systematic meta-analyses.

5. Method

5.1. EBP-group

The review of research within the field of early communication intervention that is presented in this study was initiated by the Swedish association of Habilitation directors as part of a project concerning EBP that was started 2002. Within the frames of this project several reports have been produced with respect to interventions for children and adults with disability. The author of this chapter was appointed scientific leader for a group of five speech-language pathologists and one special educator in Sweden, that applied for taking part in the project. The group has worked together during recurrent two-day-sessions and in between, work has also been done separately and in pairs.

5.2. EBP-method and search question

The group decided to use the EBP-model of Ralph Schlosser [49]. As mentioned above the hierarchy of evidence of Schlosser is a bit different compared to the traditional ones, in that it places the meta-analysis on top of the hierarchy beside the RCT-study. Schlosser also includes perspectives of the stakeholder and the influence of environment into his model of EBP and defines EBP as follows: "The integration of best and current research evidence with clinical/educational expertise and relevant stakeholder perspectives to facilitate decisions for assessment and intervention that are deemed effective and efficient for a given stakeholder". The classical model of formulation of a evidence question shortened PICO - Problem, Intervention, Comparison, Outcome - has accordingly been revised into PESICO - Problem, Environment, Stakeholders, Intervention, Comparison, Outcome [49]. The question that was formulated in this review was: A young child with severe communicative disability, living with his/her parents and being placed in a pree-school group: which intervention is most effective; indirect or direct interventions.

5.3. Procedure

When the clinical question had been formulated the group identified search terms to use. These were: Early Intervention, Communication, Communication Disability/ies, Direct intervention, Indirect intervention, Early childhood, Kindergarten, Pree-school, AAC, Augmentative Communication, Alternative Communication, Early Communication, Language, Meta-analysis, Review. The terms were searched separately and in combinations using four scientific data bases: PubMed, PsycInfo, CINAHL and ERIC. It was seen that CINAHL generated significantly more results than the other three. All abstract were browsed and the studies considered as relevant were downloaded. The reference lists of these studies led to some new findings. A few studies and book chapters were found through the group's different contacts and readings of literature. The studies were read and reviewed using a protocol and a manual that was developed. The factors that were examined in each study were: Research methods, participants, environment, intervention, results, evidence grading and a final category called notes. This column included judgements of (a) ICF domain/s that the study involved, (b) validity: internal, external, social and ecological, (c) importance of discussion and suggestions of future studies.

Each study was first reviewed by two group members separately and then discussed and graded by the group altogether. The group graded the studies according to three systems: Schlosser [49], Nordenström [51] and Golper [52]. Schlosser's system was seen as the most important for this study due to the fact that it was developed for the field of communication intervention for people with disability. Nordenström represent the classical medical evidence hierarchy whilst the Golper was included for its ambition to catch or grade the level or depth of evaluation that the study represents.

System	Level	Definition
Schlosser	1	Meta-analyses of SSRD /RCT
	2	Well designed non-RCT group study SSRD – one intervention SSRD – several interventions Subgroups to/variants of the types above
	3	Narrative quantitative reviews (except of meta-analyses)
	4	Narrative reviews
	5	Pre- experimental group studies (i.e. before-after) and case studies
	6	Expertise: educational books, journals, expert opinion
Nordenström	A	Strong scientific evidence (meta-analysis, well-done and large RCT)
	B	Moderate evidence (smaller or non-randomized studies, cross-sectional studies, case studies, cohort studies)
	C	Week evidence (expert opinion, concensus reports, case studies and other descriptive reports)
	D	Non-existent scientific evidence (No studies of sufficient quality exists).
Golper	Phase I	Hypotheses about treatment efficacy are being developed for later testing. Often this involves experimental manipulations to test potential benefits or activity of a particular treatment.
	Phase II	The goals are to formulate and standardize protocols, validate measurement instruments, optimise dosage of treatment, and so on. Includes case reports and small group studies with no control groups or treatment comparisons.
	Phase III	Treatment efficacy of a specified protocol is formally tested either with SSRD or group studies with controls such as control groups or treatment comparisons.

Table 1. Systems for evidence-grading being used in this study. SSRD=Singel Subject Research Design, RCT=Randomized Controlled Study

Author&year	Study design	Intervention	Evidence grading
Aldred, Green & Adams, 2004 [54]	RCT	Education and guidance of parents in the use of responsive strategies	Schlosser: 1 Nordenström Golper. III
Callenberg och Ganebratt, 2009 [56]	Pre-experimental group-study	ComAlong parental education; responsive strategies and AAC	Schlosser: 5 Nordenström: B Golper. II
Drew, Baird, Baron-Cohen, Cox, Slonims, Wheelwright, Swettenham, Berry & Charman, 2002 [32]	Pilot RCT	Focus parent training; joint attention	Schlosser: 1 Nordenström: A Golper. III
Elder, Valcante, Yarandi, White & Elder, 2005 [57]	Large-scale SSRD	Education and guidance of fathers: imitation and responsive strategies	Schlosser: 2 Nordenström: B Golper. III
Ferm, Andersson, Broberg, Liljegren & Thunberg, 2011 [55]	Group study; mixed methods	Parents and course leaders' experiences of the ComAlong augmentative and alternative communication early intervention course	Schlosser: 5 Nordenström: B Golper. II
Girolametto, Sussman & Weitzmann, 2007 [58]	Case study, Interaction analyses	Hanen More than Words parental education and guidance: responsive strategies	Schlosser: 5 Nordenström: C Golper. III
Howlin, Gordon, Pascoe, Wade & Charman, 2007 [59]	RCT	PECS – training of pree-school teachers (and also some older children)	Schlosser: 1 Nordenström: A Golper. III
Jonsson, Kristoffersson, Ferm & Thunberg, 2011 [40]	Pre-experimental group study; mixed methods	ComAlong parental education; responsive strategies and AAC	Schlosser: 5 Nordenström: B Golper. II
Karlsson & Melltorp, 2006 [62]	Pilot group study, mixed methods	ComAlong parental education; responsive strategies and AAC	Schlosser: 5 Nordenström: B Golper. I
Lennartsson och Sörensson, 2010 [60]	Group study, small control group	ComAlong parental education; responsive strategies and AAC	Schlosser: 5 Nordenström: B Golper. II
McConachie, Randle, Hammal & LeCouteur, 2005 [61]	Controlled group study	Hanen More than Words parental education and guidance: responsive strategies	Schlosser: 2 Nordenström: B Golper: III
Oosterling et al., 2010 [63]	RCT	Focus parent training; joint attention	Schlosser: 1 Nordenström: A Golper. III
Seung, Ashwell, Elder & Valcante, 2006 [64]	Group study	Verbal outcomes after training of fathers as analyzed by video interactions	Schlosser: 2 Nordenström: B Golper. III
Sharry, Guerin, Griffin & Drumm, 2005 [65]	Group study	Evaluation of the parental plus progam including responsive strategies	Schlosser: 5 Nordenström: B Golper. II

Table 2. Studies of education and guidance to parents or staff

The results were analysed and grouped primarily according to the formulated search question but also according to the identified areas of intervention and methods being evaluated in the studies. Building on these results, recommendations and a model for early communicative intervention was suggested. These results were documented in a report being published on the website of the Association of Swedish Habilitation directors [53]. A new literature search using the same procedure as described above led to some revision of results and recommendations in a new version of the report that was recently published [53].

The results that will be shared in this book chapter concerns the studies that specifically involved children on the autism spectrum, which in total involved about half of the studies, or exactly 47 studies. The data from both literature searches was used: 30 studies from the review published in 2011 and 16 studies from the updated version of 2012.

6. Results

The number of studies that were included in the review totalled 106. Of these, 39 were reviews, while the other 67 were primary studies. 46 of the studies involved children diagnosed within the autism spectrum. This means that about half the research on interventions for children with communicative disabilities have focused children with ASD. 31 of the studies were included in the report published 2011 while 14 were added in the review done 2012. 20 of the publications were reviews while 27 were primary studies. There were comparatively more primary studies, often of high research quality, to be found in the more recent search (2012). Only publications where the children were clearly described as having ASD were included in this review. There were most probably even more studies of the 106 that included children with ASD since sometimes participants were described according to type and/or severity of disability (such as severe communicative disability), and not diagnose..

6.1. Indirect interventions — Education and guidance to parents

14 primary studies were found. The evidence is moderately to strong since there are also some studies with a high level of scientific control. Many of the studies were noted as showing high validity with respect to external validity as well as social and ecological validity. In several studies the parents were involved in the evaluation procedure and measures of natural interactions were included.

In general the results of education and guidance to parents and staff are very positive although this review shows that there seems to be a lack of research when it comes to education and guidance of staff. Only one study was found where pree-school teachers were educated and guided how to use the PECS-method [32]. The results of the parental interventions indicate that they are effective in that positive results can be seen very quickly with respect to different areas and with comparatively little amount of intervention. This is also probably one of the reasons behind the trend that parental education seems to be included as a part of the more recently developed intervention programs. In the second literature search in this study more interventions were found that included guidance of parents (for example 31, 63, 74, 75, 81). Several of these interventions included education that was combined with home-visits when the therapist interacted with and trained the child during natural play situations. The parents observed these play activities and the therapist's use of behavioural strategies, which were then discussed an practiced during the sessions. The results of these comprehensive programs are included in the section of direct interventions below (table 3), but it is important to also recognize the fairly large amount of indirect instruction in these programs.

In several studies of the interventions more specifically aimed at parental education, it was seen that the parent's use of responsive strategies increased [54, 58, 60, 61, 62] and some studies showed that interaction between the parent and the child was positively affected [57, 58, 62, 65]. Some studies report that the development of communication and language in the child seems to be increased when the parents are provided with education and guidance [32, 54, 56, 61, 62, 64]. Several studies have tried to measure parental stress and other family related parameters that are expected to be affected, also out from parental interviews [54, 55, 56, 61, 65]. Most studies failed in proving effects in this respect, at least on a level of statistical significance. In some studies the researchers speculate that the questionnaires given before and after an intervention seems to fail in catching an effect. In qualitative studies parents report that they can see the problems of the child more clearly after the course and can be more open about the family problems [55]. This means that items related to family issues even might "get worse" comparing questionnaires filled in blindly before-after intervention.

So far very little is known of the long-term effects of indirect intervention. The few studies with this focus show that the effects seem to fade over time. Both clinicians and researchers hypothesize that there probably is a need to do follow-ups and/or provide booster interventions to maintain the intervention effects over time. There are also indications that the effects of a parental education on the development of the child seems to be further enhanced when the education is complemented with direct intervention to the child.

6.2. Direct interventions — Provision of training of the child

19 studies were found of which 10 were reviews (1 meta-analysis) and the rest primary studies. The scientific level of evidence varies, but the recently published primary studies being of high quality certainly strengthen evidence in the area of direct communication intervention.

Direct interventions or training of the child has proved to have a positive impact on the development of the child with ASD as is stated in most, but not so sure in all, of the studies in the table. Exactly what is described to be affected differs in different studies, depending on the focus of the study, but to a large extent also on what have been measured in a particular study. It is more common that classical didactic programs report outcomes within the function- or activity-domain, often by the use of measures of intelligence (IQ) or language (different language tests). The child-directed naturalistic interventions more often describe outcomes in terms of activity or participation and use data of communication or interaction from video analyses, parental questionnaires and interviews.

Author&year	Study design	Intervention	Evidence grading
Charman, 2010 [76]	Review	Review of developmental approaches to understanding and treating autism	Schlosser: 4 Nordenström: C Golper. I
Corsello, 2005 [66]	Review	Review and discussion of interventions 0-3 years	Schlosser: 4 Nordenström: C Golper. I
Dawson et al, 2010 [30]	RCT	Study of the effects of : The Early Start Denver Model for toddlers with ASD	Schlosser: 1 Nordenström: A Golper. III
Delprato, 2001 [67]	Review	Comparison of discrete trial interventions and naturalistic language interventions	Schlosser: 4 Nordenström: B Golper. II
Diggle & McConachie, 2009 [68]	Review Cochrane-report	Review of parent-mediated intervention/ training of children with ASD	Schlosser: 3 Nordenström: B Golper. III
Fernell et al, 2011 [77]	Comparative group study	Comparison of effects of 1) intensity and form of intervention 2) intelligence on adaptive behaviour on children with ASD	Schlosser: 2 Nordenström: B Golper. II-III
Goldstein, 2002 [69]	Review	Review and comparison of communication intervention to children with ASD	Schlosser: 4 Nordenström: B Golper. II
Kasari et al (2010) [31]	RCT	Study of the outcomes of an intervention for joint attention	Schlosser: 1 Nordenström: A Golper: III
Kasari, Paparella & Freeman, 2008 [70]	Randomized group study	Comparison of interventions for play and joint attention in children with ASD	Schlosser: 2 Nordenström: A Golper. III
McConkey et al, (2010) [74]	Controlled group study	Evaluation of the impact of home-based intervention to promote communication	Schlosser: 2 Nordenström: B Golper. III
McConnell, 2002 [71]	Review	Review of interventions to promote social interaction in young children in educational settings	Schlosser: 4 Nordenström: B Golper. I
Paul & Roth , 2011 [78]	Narrative review/ expertise	Characterizing and Predicting Outcomes of Communication Delays in Infants and Toddlers: Implications for Clinical Practice.	Schlosser: 6 Nordenström: C Golper. I
Rogers, 2006 [11]	Review	Review of and historic description of communication intervention to young children with ASD	Schlosser: 6 Nordenström: C Golper. I
Schuit et al, 2011 [79]	Controlled group study (small groups)	Evaluation of a program aimed at stimulate language learning in disabled children	Schlosser: 5 Nordenström: B Golper. III
Spreckley & Boyd, 2009 [80]	Meta-analysis	Meta-analysis of discrete-trial-interventions for children with ASD	Schlosser: 1 Nordenström: A Golper. III

Author&year	Study design	Intervention	Evidence grading
Vismara et al, 2009 [81]	Group study Non-concurrent multiple baseline design	Evaluation of the effects of "start-kit" of 12 individual sessions teaching parents communicative strategies	Schlosser: 2 Nordenström: B Golper. I
Wong & Kwang, 2010 [75]	RCT (small groups)	Evaluation of Autism 1-2-3-progam	Schlosser: 1 Nordenström: B Golper. III
Woods & Wetherby, 2003 [72]	Review, clinical report	Review of methods of identification and intervention for young children at risk of ACD	Schlosser: 4 Nordenström: C Golper. II
Yoder & Stone, 2006 [73]	Randomized comparison	Comparison of RPMT and PECS on spoken communication	Schlosser: 2 Nordenström: B Golper. III

Table 3. Studies of direct interventions and comprehensive programs

As mentioned in earlier paragraphs generalization and maintenance has been a big issue within the field of communication and language intervention for years. Generally the child-focused interventions show better generalization and maintenance in younger children with ASD [67, 72, 76]. These studies discuss that the use of the inborn motivation of the child and the use of natural context and natural play context make the difference – all according to current theories of development of cognition and communication. Proponents of didactic training hold that the use of learned words and phrases might be a start of a positive social spiral where the child gets more response and is treated differently. Some reviews come to the conclusion that we still do not have enough evidence to tell which type of program is best, didactic or child-focused, but that the important factors seem to be early start and intensity [66, 69]. According to the meta-analysis of six RCT studies of didactic interventions [80] these however fail in reporting better outcomes than the control groups when it comes to cognition, language and adaptive functioning. Generally the children in didactic training programs also were older [68]. Didactic training in its intensive and comprehensive form seems less effective on younger children and children at early communicative levels [77]. The involvement of the parents in recurrent didactic training activities in the home is also questioned in some studies [68]. There are indications of a high degree of stress in these parents and a comparative study showed that parental stress was lowered when the training was done by others and furthermore that the results with respect to communication development was enhanced [68].

Several recent studies report outcomes from eclectic comprehensive interventions [30, 31, 74]. These programs are built upon current theories of cognitive, communicative and neurophysiological development but also adds knowledge from the behaviourist tradition or rather Applied Behavior Analysis (ABA) in optimizing the learning situation. More concretely this means that these programs are child-focused in that it makes use of the child's motivation and interests and focus the communication between the parent and the child and are often implemented in the home setting, sometimes after some introductory sessions on a clinic. An analysis of the child's communication development forms the decision of what is going to be focused during interaction. Prelinguistic competencies such as imitation, joint attention and use of symbol play and symbols are seen as basic and pivotal. The behavioural techniques are used to arrange the environment and chose strategies to refine and enhance learning in the natural interaction. The trainer serve as model to the parent and then guide and coach the parent, often in the home.

The majority of the primary studies in the table above report excellent outcomes [30, 31 70, 73, 74, 75, 81]. In general the research quality of evaluations of these interventions were high since many were of RCT type or Randomized Group studies. External, social and ecological validity was also considered as generally high partly due to the use of more interactional data and information from the stakeholders. The studies show that these interventions seem to be very effective in proving positive outcomes with respect to interaction, parental communication style and child development. Some of these intervention programs are of comparatively low intensity and short, which is interesting and important, as high intensity traditionally have been said to be essential to success in children with autism

Some articles compare interventions and discuss recommendations with respect to different needs of the child or family. A comparison of the AAC-method PECS and RPMT (a comprehenesive program containing parental education in the use of responsive strategies and training of the child and guidance to parents in their home) showed interesting results with respect to communication outcomes in the children [73]. The children at the earliest communicative stage, not yet being interested in objects, seem to develop more with RPMT. At the next communicative stage when the children has an interest of objects, an understanding of cause and effect and some emergent understanding of joint attention PECS is more effective. When joint attention is more established the Prelinguistic Mileu Teching strategies (behavioral techniques implemented in natural interaction) in the RPMT seems to be more operant. It was also seen that the PMT-training had better effect for those children whose mothers used a responsive communication style. The focus on development of joint attention is emphasized as the primary goal in this study with a successive introduction of symbol play as joint attention is being established [73].

Finally, one review studies the effect of different types of interventions to promote social interaction in pree-school settings and conclude that there is good evidence that it is important to work both with the child with disability as well as with his/her friends in the school environment [71].

6.3. AAC intervention

The field of AAC is a fairly new field of knowledge that has gradually grown as there is a increasing interest in functional communication and in ensuring the communicative rights of individuals with disability. There has also been an explosion of available communication technologies and methods that can support and improve communication for individuals with autism. We have probably and hopefully only seen the dawn of these new options. It is also possible to see that we are moving from using one technique or approach at the time to working with multimodal techniques or approaches where different tools and methods combined with an understanding of communication and use of interactional strategies build a total system of communication.

Author&year	Study design	Intervention	Evidence grading
Binger, Berens, Kent-Walsh &Taylor, 2008 [82]	Review	The impact of AAC-intervention on use of AAC, symbolic gestures and speech	Schlosser: 4 Nordenström: B Golper. II
Bopp, Brown & Mirenda, 2004 [83]	Review	Review of FCT and use of visual strategies and discussion of the role of speech-language pathologist in working with challenging behaviors	Schlosser: 4 Nordenström: B Golper. I
Brady, 2000 [84]	Case study	Study of the impact of use of SGDs on the understanding of speech	Schlosser: 5 Nordenström: C Golper. I
Branson & Demcak, 2009 [85]	Meta-analysis	Evaluation of AAC interventions for toddlers and infants with disability	Schlosser: 1 Nordenström: A Golper. III
Ganz, Simpson & Corbin-Newsome, 2008 [86]	SSRD – Multiple baseline	Impact of PECS on requesting and speech	Schlosser: 2 Nordenström: B Golper. III
Mancil et al(2009) [95]	SSRD – multiple baseline	Study of the effects of a picture-exhange-intervention using milieu teaching in the home	Schlosser: 2 Nordenström: B Golper. III
Millar, Light & Schlosser 2006 [87]	Meta-analysis	The impact of AAC-interventions on speech development	Schlosser: 1 Nordenström: B Golper. I
Papparella & Kasari, 2004 [88]	Review	Study of the relationship between joint attention and language – manual signing	Schlosser:4 Nordenström: C Golper. I
Preston & Carter, 2009 [89]	Meta-analysis	Study of the effects of PECS	Schlosser: 1 Nordenström: B Golper. III
Schlosser &, 2006 [90]	Quantitative review	The impact of AAC on children with developmental disabilites	Schlosser: 4 Nordenström: B Golper. II
Schlosser & Wendt, 2008 [91]	Meta-analysis	Effects of different types of AAC on speech in children with ASD	Schlosser: 1 Nordenström: B Golper: II
Sigafoos, Drasgow, Reichle, O´Reilly & Tait, 2004 [92]	Review	Study of the effectiveness of training of rejecting using AAC	Schlosser: 4 Nordenström: B Golper. I
Snell, Chen, Lih-Huan & Hoover, 2006 [94]	Review	Review of AAC-interventions to children with severe communicative disabilities	Schlosser: 4 Nordenström: B Golper. I
van der Meer et al, 2011 [93]	Controlled group study	Evaluation of a program using AAC (not further described)	Schlosser: 5 Nordenström: B Golper. II

Table 4. Studies of education and guidance to parents

The research base with respect to AAC used by young children with autism has grown in recent years. This research mostly consists of singe-subject-design studies and case studies, with very few controlled group studies being done. On the other hand there are some well-done meta-analyses published that compile results from singe-subject research studies. Due to the difficulties of conducting RCT studies within the field of AAC-intervention the meta-anlyses are important and can be seen as the golden standard. In total 14 studies were identified as focusing the use of AAC and of these 10 were reviews or meta-analyses.

In conclusion, meta-analyses and other studies show that AAC-interventions are cost-effective and give fast results and furthermore tend to stimulate speech development [82, 84, 85, 86, 87, 91]. The best results seem to be reached when the social network surrounding a child is given support and resources, to be able to use responsive strategies and provide communication opportunities and direct training using AAC in natural daily interactions. AAC intervention should be started as soon as communication difficulties are displayed or suspected since AAC promotes communication, language and speech. AAC-intervention has also been proved to effectively decrease challenging behaviour [83]. There is today no mode of AAC that is known to be better than any other for young children with autism. Instead multimodal approaches seem to be the most effective [93]. However, graphic AAC seem to be acquired at a faster rate and also easier to generalize to other situations [90]. PECS has been proved to be an effective AAC method, specifically at early stages of communication and with respect to the first three phases of the method [89].

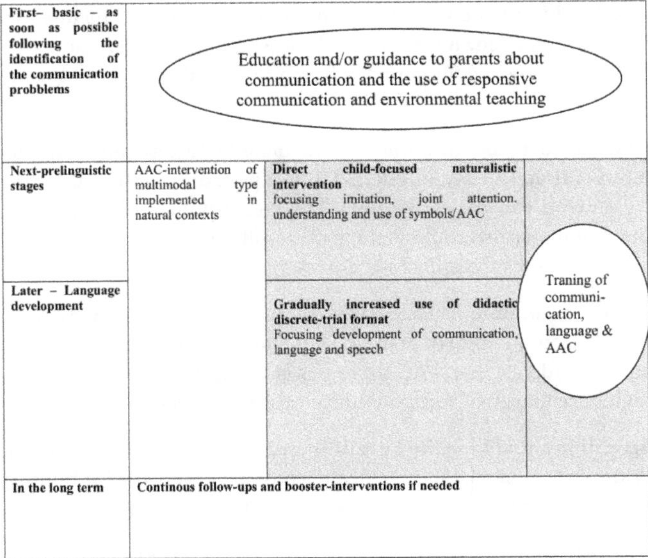

Figure 1. Model for early communication intervention

7. Conclusion

The conclusion of this chapter is presented in the form of eight recommendations and of a model for early communication intervention answering the question that was initially formulated in this study: **"A young child with autism and severe communicative disability, living with his/her parents and being placed in a pree-school group: which intervention is most effective; indirect or direct interventions?"**

1. **A combination of indirect and direct interventions.** There is strong evidence that the combination of education and guidance to the parents and direct child-focused intervention to the child in a naturalistic context leads to good outcomes with respect to several parameters such as: development of communication and language, interaction between the parent and the child where the parent uses a responsive communication pattern,

2. **Parental education should include knowledge of and training in the use of responsive strategies and behavioural/environmental teaching techniques within the frames of natural interaction in the home.** Several studies show that parents change their communicative style after a few education sessions and that this positively affect the interaction pattern with the child and enhance language development in the child. **Guidance or coaching of the parents in natural interactions in the home environment** is included in most of the recently presented studies and show very good results in short time.

3. **Direct interventions provided to children on early communicative stage should be child-focused and implemented in daily natural interactions. The intervention should focus imitation, joint attention and symbol use** (speech, symbols, manual signs). Didactic intervention is not effective for young children since maintenance and generalization of training is low.

4. **Interventions need to be continuous and include follow-ups and possibilities of booster-intervention.** The few long-term follow up-studies all show that interventions (of different type) tend to wear off by time. The recent published studies show that low-intensity interventions also could yield good results. The engagement of the parent also might be an important success factor.

5. **Children at early communicative stages should be provided with AAC as early as possible.** There is no age-limit or prerequisites that need to met before AAC is introduced. There is strong evidence that AAC decreases challenging behaviour. There is moderate to strong evidence that AAC facilitates development of speech.

6. **AAC-intervention should ideally be multimodal.** All modes of AAC are effective. There is some evidence that symbols (specifically combined with speech output) are learned faster than manual signs and that iconic symbols are learned faster.

7. **PECS (Picture Exchange Communication System) is an effective AAC-method for children at early communicative stages.** There is strong evidence that PECS has a positive effect on interaction and behaviour and that functional communication is increased.

8. **The AAC-modes should be used and modelled by the child's communication partners** (aided language stimulation or modelling) to promote learning and spontaneous use of the symbols.

These recommendations means that the child in our formulated question should be provided with intervention according to the model below.

Acknowledgements

Parts of chapter two, three and four was first published in the author's thesis [96]. Thanks to my collegues in the ebp-group: Lena Nilsson, Maria Nolemo, Barbara Eberhart, Jessica Forsberg, Ruth Breivik and Anna Fäldt.

Author details

Gunilla Thunberg*

DART – Centre for AAC and Assistive Technology, Sahlgrenska University Hospital, Sweden

References

[1] Short C, Schopler E. Factors relating to age of onset in autism. Journal of Autism and Developmental Disorders 1988 ;18 207–216.

[2] Carr EG, Levin L, McConnachie G, Carlson JI, Kemp DC, Smith CE. Communication-based intervention for problem behavior. Baltimore, MD: Paul H. Brookes Publishing; 1997.

[3] Billstedt E. Children with autism grow up: Use of the DISCO (Diagnostic Interview for Social and COmmunication disorders) in population cohorts. Göteborg: Göteborg University; 2007.

[4] Billstedt E, Gillberg IC, Gillberg C. Autism after adolescence: Population-based 13-22-year follow-up study of 120 individuals with autism diagnosed in childhood. Journal of Autism and Developmental Disorders 2005 ; 35, 351–360.

[5] Howlin P, Goode S, Hutton J, Rutter M. Adult outcomes for children with autism. Journal of Child Psychology and Psychiatry, 2004; 45, 212–229.

[6] Shea V, Mesibov G. Adolescents and adults with autism. In F. Volkmar, R. Paul, A. Klin & D. Cohen (Eds.), Handbook of autism and pervasive developmental disorders (pp. 288–311). Hoboken, NJ: John Wiley & Sons; 2005.

[7] Bryson S. Brief report: Epidemiology of autism. Journal of Autism and Developmental Disorders 1996; 26, 165–167.

[8] Bryson S, Clark BS, Smith TM. First report of a Canadian epidemiological study of autistic syndromes. Journal of Child Psychology and Psychiatry 1988; 29, 433–445.

[9] Lord C, Risi S, Pickles. Trajectory of language development in autism spectrum disorders. In R. M & S. Warren (Eds.), Developmental language disorders: From phenotypes to etiologies (pp. 7–29). Mahwah, NJ: Lawrence Erlbaum; 2004.

[10] Tager-Flusberg H., Joseph RM. Identifying neurocognitive phenotypes in autism. Philosophical Transactions of the Royal Society of London, Series B: Biological Sciences 2003; 358, 303–314.

[11] Rogers S. Evidence-based interventions for language development in young children with autism. In T. Charman & W. Stone (Eds.) Social and communication development in autism spectrum disorders (pp. 143–179). New York: The Guildford Press ; 2006.

[12] Tager-Flusberg H, Paul R, Lord C. Language and communication in autism. In F. Volkmar, R. Paul, A. Klin & D. Cohen (Eds.) Handbook of autism and pervasive developmental disorders (Vol. 1, pp. 335–364). Hoboken, NJ: John Wiley & Sons ; 2005.

[13] Wetherby A M, Prizant BM, Schuler AL. Understanding the nature of communication and language impairments. In AM Wetherby & BM Prizant (Eds.), Autism spectrum disorders: A transactional developmental perspective pp. 109–141. Baltimore, MD: Paul H. Brookes Publishing; 2000.

[14] Tager-Flusberg H, Joseph R, Folstein S. Current directions in research on autism. Mental Retardation and Developmental Disabilities Research Reviews 2001; 7, 21–29.

[15] Wetherby AM. Understanding and measuring social communication in children with autism spectrum disorders. In T. Charman & W. Stone (Eds.*), Social and communication development in autism spectrum disorders* (pp. 3–34). New York: The Guildford Press: 2006.

[16] Charman T, Baron-Cohen S, Swettenham J, Baird G, Drew A, Cox A. Predicting language outcome in infants with autism and pervasive developmental disorder. International Journal of Language and Communication Disorders 2003; 38, 265–285.

[17] Mundy P, Sigman M, Kasari C. A longitudinal study of joint attention and language development in autistic children. Journal of Speech and Hearing Research 1990; 38, 157–167.

[18] Dahlgren SO, Gillberg C. Symptoms in the first two years of life: A preliminary population study of infantile autism. European Archives of Psychiatric and Neurological Science 1989; 283, 169–174.

[19] Osterling J, Dawson G. Early recognition of children with autism: A study of first birthday home videotapes. Journal of Autism and Developmental Disorders 1994; 24, 247–258.

[20] Watson LR, Baranek GT, Crais ER, Reznick SJ, Dykstra J, Perryman T. The first year inventory: Retrospective parent responses to a questionnaire designed to identify one-year olds at risk for autism. Journal of Autism and Developmental Disorders 2007: 37, 49–61.

[21] Chawarska K, Paul R, Klin A, Hannigen S, Dichtel L E, Volkmar F. Parental recognition of developmental problems in toddlers with autism spectrum disorders. Journal of Autism and Developmental Disorders 2007; 37, 62–72.

[22] Lord C, Schulman C, DiLavore P. Regression and word loss in autistic spectrum disorders. Journal of Child Psychology and Psychiatry 2004; 45, 936–955.

[23] Wetherby AM. Ontogeny of communicative functions in autism. Journal of Autism and Developmental Disorders 1986; 16, 295–316.

[24] Ramberg C, Ehlers S, Nydén A, Johansson M, Gillberg C. Language and pragmatic functions in school-age children on the autism spectrum. European Journal of Disorders of Communication 1996; 31, 387–413.

[25] Bishop D, Hartley J, Weir F. Why and when do some language-impaired children seem talkative? A study of initiation in conversation of children with semantic-pragmatic disorders. Journal of Autism and Developmental Disorders 1994 ; 24, 177–197.

[26] Lovaas OI, Koegel RL, Simmons JQ, Long JS. Some generalization and follow-up measures on autistic children in behaviour therapy. Journal of Applied Behavior Analysis 1973; 6, 131–166.

[27] Hart BM, Risley TR. Establishing use of descriptive adjectives in the spontaneous speech of disadvantaged preschool children. Journal of Applied Behavior Analysis 1968; 1, 109–120.

[28] Prizant BM, Wetherby AM, Rydell P. Communication intervention issues for children with autism spectrum disorders. In A. M. Wetherby & B. M. Prizant (Eds.), Autism spectrum disorders: A transactional developmental perspective. Baltimore, MD: Paul H. Brookes Publishing; 2000.

[29] Hancock TB, Kaiser AP. The effects of trainer-implemented enhanced milieu-teaching on the social communication of children with autism. Topics in Early Childhood Special Education 2002; 22, 29–54.

[30] Dawson G, Rogers S, Munson J, Smith M, Winter J, Greenson J, Donaldson A, Varley J. Randomized, Controlled Trial of an Intervention for Toddlers With Autism: The Early Start Denver Model. Pediatrics 2010; 125; e17.

[31] Kasari C, Gulsrud AC, Wong C, Kwon S, Locke J. Randomized controlled caregiver mediated joint engagement intervention for toddlers with autism. Journal of Autism and Developmental disorders 2010; 40, 1045-1056.

[32] Drew A, Baird G, Baron-Cohen S, Cox A, Slonims V, Wheelwright S, Swettenham J, Berry B, Charman T. A pilot randomised control trial of a parent training intervention for pre-school children with autism: preliminary findings and methodological challenges. European Child & Adolescent Psychiatry 2002; 11(6) s. 266-272.

[33] Dahlgren S, Dahlgren-Sandberg A. The non-specificity of theory of mind deficits: Evidence from children with communicative disabilities. European Journal of Cognitive psychology 2004; 15, 129-155.

[34] Ello LM, Donovan SJ. Assessment of the relationship between parenting stress and a child's ability to functionally communicate. Research on Social Work Practice 2005;15(6), 531-544.

[35] Wilder J, Granlund M. Behaviour style and interaction between seven children with multiple disabilities and their caregivers. Child: care, health and development 2003; 29, 559-567.

[36] Warren S, Brady N, Sterling A, Fleming K, Marquis J. Maternal responsivity predicts language development in young children with fragile X syndrome. American Journal on Intellectual Disabilities 2010;115 (1), 54-75.

[37] Siller M, Sigman M. The behaviors of parents of children with autism predict the subsequent development of their children's communication. Journal of Autism and Developmental Disorders 2002; 32, 77-89.

[38] Hanen centre. http://www.hanen.org (accessed 23 October 2012).

[39] AKKtiv. http://www.akktiv.se (accessed 23 October 2012).

[40] Jonsson A, Kristoffersson L, Ferm U, Thunberg G. The ComAlong communication boards: Parents' use and experiences of aided language stimulation. Augmentative and Alternative Communication 2011; 27 (2), 103–116.

[41] Howlin P. Augmentative and alternative communication systems for children with autism. InT. Charman & W. Stone (Eds.), Social and communication development in autism spectrum disorders (pp. 236–266). New York: The Guildford Press: 2006.

[42] Mirenda P, Erickson KA. Augmentative communication and literacy. In B. M. Prizant & A. M. Wetherby (Eds.), Autism spectrum disorders: A transactional developmental perspective (pp. 369–394). Baltimore, MD: Paul H. Brookes Publishing. 2000.

[43] Yoder PJ, Layton TL. Speech following sign language training in autistic children with minimal verbal language. Journal of Autism and Developmental Disorders 1988: 18, 217–230.

[44] Seal BC, Bonvillian JD. Sign language and motor functioning in students with autistic disorders. Journal of Autism and Developmental Disorders 1997; 27, 437–466.

[45] Schopler E, Reichler R, Lansing M. Teaching strategies for parents and professionals. Austin, TX: PRO-ED Inc: 1980.

[46] Danielsson H, Jönsson, B. Pictures as language. Paper presented at the International Conference on Language and Visualisation, Stockholm: 2001.

[47] Bondy A, Frost L. The Picture Exchange Communication System. Focus on Autistic Behavior, 1994: 9, 1–19.

[48] Schlosser RW, Blischak DM. Is there a role for speech output in interventions for persons with autism. Focus on Autism and Other Developmental Disabilities 2001;16, 170–176.

[49] Schlosser RW. The Efficacy of Augmentative and Alternative Communication: Towards Evidence-Based Practice. Baltimore: Paul Brookes: 2003.

[50] Schlosser RW, Raghavendra P. Evidence-Based Practice in Augmentative andAlternative Communication. Augmentative and Alternative Communication 2004; 20, 1-21.

[51] Nordenström J. Evidensbaserad medicin: I Sherlock Holmes fotspår. Stockholm: Karolinska University Press; 2006.

[52] Golper LAC, Wertz RT, Frattali CM, Yorkston K, Myers P, Katz.R, Beeson P, Kennedy MRT, Bayles K, Wambaugh J. Evidence-based practice guidelines for the management of communication disorders inneurologically impaired individuals: Project introduction. ANCDS: 2001.

[53] Sveriges habiliteringschefer [Swedish habilitation directors]. http://www.sverigeshabiliteringschefer.se (accessed 23 october 2012).

[54] Aldred C, Green J, Adams C. A new social intervention for children with autism: pilot randomised controlled treatment study suggesting effectiveness. Journal of Child Psychology and Psychiatry 2004;45(1) 1420-1430.

[55] Ferm U, Andersson M, Broberg M, Liljegren T, Thunberg G. Parents and course leaders' experiences of the ComAlong augmentative and alternative communication early intervention course. Disability Studies Quarterly: Mediated Communication 2011; 31(4) http://dsq-sds.org

[56] Callenberg A, Ganebratt P. Utvärdering av AKKtiv föräldrautbildning: föräldrars bedömningar av barnens kommunikativa utveckling. [Evaluation of ComAlong parental course: parents' views and development in children]. Unpublished masters' thesis in Speech-language Pathology, University of Gothenburg: Department of Neuroscience and Physiology, Gothenburg: 2009.

[57] Elder JH, Valcante G, Yarandi H, White D, Elder TH. Evaluating In-Home Training for Fathers of Children With Autism Using Single-Subject Experimentation and Group Analysis Methods. Nursing Research 2009; vol 54 no 1.

[58] Girolametto L, Sussman F, Weitzmann E. Using case study methods to investigate the effects of interactive intervention for children with autism spectrum disorders. Journal of Communication Disorders 2007; 40, 470-492.

[59] Howlin P, Gordon K, Pasco G, Wade A, Charman T. The effectiveness of Picture Exchange Communication System (PECS) training for teachers of children with autism: a pragmatic, group randomised controlled trial. J Child Psychol Psychiatry. 2007; 48(5):473-81.

[60] Lennartsson E, Sörensson K. Föräldrars sätt att kommunicera med sina barn före och efter Komlgång kommunikationskurs. [Parental communication style before and after ComAlong parental course]. Unpublished masters' thesis in Speech-language Pathology, University of Gothenburg: Department of Neuroscience and Physiology, Gothenburg: 2010.

[61] McConachie H, Randle V, Hammal D, Le Couteur A. A controlled trial of training course for parents of children with suspected autism spectrum disorders. The Journal of Pediatrics 2005; 14, 335-40.

[62] Karlsson E, Melltorp M. Utvärdering av AKKtiv: Tidig intervention till föräldrar som har barn med omfattande kommunikationssvårigheter. [Evaluation of ComAlong: Early intervention to parents of children with communicative disability]. Unpublished masters' thesis in Speech-language Pathology, University of Gothenburg: Department of Neuroscience and Physiology, Gothenburg: 2006.

[63] Oosterling I, Visser J, Swinkels S, Rommelse N, Donders, R, Woudenberg T, Roos S, van der Gaag RJ, Biotelaar J. Randomized controlled trial of the Focus parent training for toddlers with autism: 1-year outcome. Journal of Autism and Developmental Disorders 2010; 40, 1447-1458.

[64] Seung HK, Ashwell S, Elder JH, Valcante G. (2006). Verbal communication outcomes in children with autism after in-home father training. Journal of Intellectual Disability Research, 2, (50), 139-150.

[65] Sharry J, Guerin S, Griffin C, Drumm, M. (2005). An evaluation of the Parents Plus Early Years Programme: A video-based early intervention for parents of pre-school children with behavioural and developmental difficulties. Clinical Child Psychology and Psychiatry, 10, 319.

[66] Corsello CM. Early Intervention in Autism. Infants & Young Children 2005; 18(2) 74-85.

[67] Delprato, D. J., (2001) Comparisons of Discrete-Trial and Normalized Behavioral Language Intervention for Young Children with Autism. Journal of Autism and Developmental Disorders, 31, 315-325.

[68] Diggle TTJ, McConachie HHR. Parent-mediated early intervention for young children with autism spectrum disorder (Review). The Cochrane Library 2009, Issue 4.

[69] Goldstein H. Communication Intervention for Children with Autism: A Review of Treatment Efficacy. Journal of Autism and Development Disorders 2002; 32(5), 373-396.

[70] Kasari C, Papparella T, Freeman S. Language Outcome in Autism: Randomized Comparison of Joint Attention and Play Interventions. Journal of Consulting and Clinical Psychology 2008; 76(1) 125-137.

[71] McConnell S. Intervention to Facilitate Social Interaction for Young Children with Autism: Review of Available Research and Recommendations for Educational Intervention and Future Research. Journal of Autism and Developmental Disorders 2002; 32(5) 351-372.

[72] Woods J, Wetherby A. Early Indentification of and Intervention for Infant and Toddlers Who Are at Risk for Autism Spectrum Disorder, Language, Speech and Hearing in Schools, 2003; 34 180-193.

[73] Yoder P. Stone WL. A Randomized Comparison of the Effect of Two Prelinguistic Communication Interventions on the Acquisition of Spoken Communication in Preschoolers With ASD. Journal of Speech, Language and Hearing Research 2006; 49 698-771.

[74] McConkey R, Truesdale-Kennedy M, Crawford H, McGreevy E, Reavey M, Cassidy A. Preeschoolers with autism spectrum disorders: evaluating the impact of home-based intervention to promote their communication. Early Child Development and Care 2010; 180(3) 299-315.

[75] Wong VCN, Kwan QK. Randomized Controlled Trial for Early Intervention for Autism: A Pilot Study of the Autism 1-2-3 Project. Journal of Developmental Disorder 2010; 40 677-688.

[76] Charman, T. (2010). Developmental Approaches to Understanding and Treating Autism. Folia Phoniatrica et Logopaedica, 62, 166-177.

[77] Fernell E, Hedvall Å, Westerlund J, Höglund Carlsson L, Eriksson M, Barnevik Olsson M, Holm A, Norrelgen F, Kjellmer L, Gillberg C. Early Intervention in 208 Swedish preschoolers with autism spectrum disorder. A prospective naturalistic study Research in developmental Disabilities 2011; 32 2092-2101.

[78] Paul R, Roth FP. Characterizing and Predicting Outcomes of Communication Delays in Infants and Toddlers: Implications for Clinical Practice. Language, Speech, and Hearing Services in Schools, 42, 331-340.

[79] Van der Schuit M, Segers E, Van Balkom H. Verhoeven L. Early language intervention for children with intellectual disabilities: A neurocognitive perspective. Research in Developmental Disabilities 2011; 32 705-712.

[80] Spreckley M, Boyd R. Efficacy of Applied Behavioural intervention in preschool children with autism for improving cognitive, language and adaptive behaviour. A systematic review and meta-analysis. J Pediatr 2009; 154 338-344.

[81] Vismara LA, Colombi C, Rogers SJ. Can one hour per week of therapy lead to lasting changes in young children with autism? Autism 2009; 13(1) 93-115.

[82] Binger C, Berens J, Kent-Walsh J, Taylor S. The Effects of Aided AAC Interventions on AAC Use, Speech, and Symbolic Gestures. Seminars och Speech and language 2008; 29 101-111.

[83] Bopp K, Brown K. Mirenda P. Speech-Language Pathologists' Roles in the Delivery of Positive Behaviour Support for Individuals With Developmental Disabilities. American Journal of Speech-Language Pathology 2004; 13 5-19.

[84] Brady NC. (2000). Improved Comprehension of Object Names Following Voice Output Communication Aid Use: Two case Studies. Augmentative and Alternative Communication, 16, 197-204.

[85] Branson D Demchak M. The use of Augmentative and Alternative Communication Methods with Infants and Toddlers with Disabilities: A Research Review. Augmentative and Alternative Communication 2009; 25 274-286.

[86] Ganz JB, Simpson RL, Corbin-Newsome J. The impact of the Picture Excange Communication System om requesting and speech development in preschoolers with autism spectrum disorders and similar characteristics. Research in Autism Spectrum Disorders 2008; 2 157-169.

[87] Millar DC, Light JC Schlosser RW. The Impact of Augmentative and Alternative Communication Intervention on the Speech Production of Individuals with Developmental Disabilities: A Research Review. Journal of Speech, Language and Hearing Research 2006; 49 248-264.

[88] Papparella T. Kasari C. Joint Attention Skills and Language Development in Special Needs Populations Translating Research to Practice. Infants and Young Children 2004; 17(3) 269–280.

[89] Preston D. Carter M. A Review of the Efficacy of the Picture Exchange Communication System Intervention. Journal of Autism and Developmental Disorders 2009; 39 1471-1486.

[90] Schlosser R. Sigafoos J. Augmentative and Alternative communication interventions for persons with developmental disabilities: narrative review of comparative single-subject experimental studies Research in Developmental Disabilities 2006; 27 1-29.

[91] Schlosser R. Wendt O. Effects of Augmentative and Alternative Communication Intervention on Speech Production in Children With Autism: A Systematic Review. American Journal of Speech-Language Pathology 2008; 17 212-223.

[92] Sigafoos J, Drasgow E, Reichle J, O'Reilly M, Green V, Tait K. Forum on Intervention Strategies for Severe Disabilities Tutorial: Teaching Communicative Rejecting to Children With Severe Disabilities. American Journal of Speech-Language Pathology 2004; 13 31-42

[93] van der Meer L, Sigafoos J, O'Reilly M. Lancioni, G. Assessing preferences for AAC options in communication interventions for individuals with developmental disabilities: A review of the literature. Research in Developmental Disabilities 2011; 32 1422–1431.

[94] Snell M, Chen L-Y & Hoover K. Teaching Augmentative and Alternative Communication to Students With Severe Disabilities: A Review of Intervention Research 1997-2003. Research and Practice for Persons with Severe Disabilities 2006; 3, 203-214.

[95] Mancil RG, Conroy AC, Haydon TF. Effects of a Modified Milieu Therapy Intervention on the Social Communicative Behaviours of Young Children with Autism Spectrum Disorders. Journal of Autism and Developmental Disorders 2009; 39 149-163.

[96] Thunberg, G. Using speech-generating devices at home. A study of children with autism spectrum disorders at different stages of communication development. Gothenburg Monographs in Linguistics 34. Göteborg, Sweden: Göteborg University: 2007.

Section 2

Aetiological Factors - The Autistic Self and Creativity

Chapter 8

Critical Evaluation of the Concept of Autistic Creativity

Viktoria Lyons and Michael Fitzgerald

Additional information is available at the end of the chapter

1. Introduction

Autism Spectrum Disorders (ASD) are neurodevelopmental conditions that are associated with an astonishing combination of cognitive strengths and weaknesses with a substantial minority of individuals displaying some exceptional creative abilities, reaching genius proportions in some rare cases. Creativity is a multifactorial construct and neuroscience is only beginning to unravel some of the cognitive components involved in the creative process. In this chapter we contrast neuroscientific evidence from creativity research with models attempting to explain talent and creativity in ASD. Although there are no agreed definitions for creativity the formulation put forward by Griffiths [1] "Creativity is a mental journey between ideas or concepts that involves either a novel route or a novel destination" (p.6) seems to fit the picture very well. Various explanations and theories have been put forward to account for creativity ranging from unconscious mechanisms, cognitive processes, special abilities and personal traits to links with genetic processes and psychopathology.

The classical portrait of autism is that of rigid, stereotyped behaviours, a preference for sameness and a resulting lack of imagination. Therefore, the prevalent view is that creativity and imaginative thought are extremely difficult or impossible for individuals with ASD. There is substantial research evidence that almost all forms of imagination are impaired in autism including lack of pretend play, pragmatic language, comprehension and construction of narrative, theory of mind and experimental tests of creativity [2-6]. A significant challenge to this perceived lack of creativity is the enormous achievements that some people with ASD show in creative and scientific fields. Some theorists and clinicians have therefore challenged the view of impoverished creativity in ASD [7-12].

In this review the focus is on a subgroup of individuals on the autistic spectrum who display exceptional creative talents and abilities. The features of ASD that favour creativity include narrow interests, great persistence, ability to see details within a whole, a fascination with facts (rather than people) and having savant type talents. While social imagination is impaired, autistic imagination of the Einsteinian type is amplified.

2. Nature of autistic intelligence and creativity

"Autistic intelligence" as described by Hans Asperger [13] is a sort of intelligence hardly touched by tradition and culture – "unconventional, unorthodox, strangely 'pure' and original, akin to the intelligence of pure creativity". As pointed out by Einstein "To raise new questions, new possibilities, to regard old problems from a new angle, requires imagination and makes real advance in science" [14 p. 40].

Individuals with ASD show great variation in IQ ranging from severe intellectual impairment to superior ability. In addition, intelligence as measured by traditional intelligence tests reveals a different intellectual profile in ASD than in the neurotypical population with peaks on Block Design and troughs in Comprehension that appears to be robust across IQ levels [15]. Individuals with ASD also generally display atypical cognitive processes when performing these tasks. More recent studies [16,17] revealed further evidence for a different nature of autistic intelligence including fast information processing despite poor measured IQ.

The relationship between intelligence and creativity is unclear and ranges from suggestions of totally distinct psychological entities to overlapping constructs to different labels for the same thing [18]. Guilford [19] in his 1950 landmark paper "Creativity" asserted that creative talent could not be understood in terms of "intelligence". Within the creativity literature, as noted by Lubart [20] "the dominant view is that certain intellectual abilities may be particularly useful in creative work, but no intellectual ability is devoted only to creativity" (p.288). Good general intelligence, domain-specific knowledge and special skills are necessary ingredients for creativity; however, these components alone are not sufficient for explaining creative processes [21].

Gardner's [22] model of multiple intelligences holds that intelligence is a collection of different intellectual capacities including linguistic, logical-mathematical, musical, bodily kinaesthetic, spatial intelligence and two forms of personal intelligence, - one oriented towards the understanding of other persons, the other towards an understanding of self. Autistic intelligence tends to be concentrated in the areas of music and logical-mathematical and spatial abilities. By nature, individuals with autism are extremely logical and analytical, and their thinking is concrete which makes them good mathematicians though lesser poets. The exception may be a minority of gifted individuals with ASD who have special literary talents as suggested by Ilona Roth [23] in her analysis of autism spectrum poets including Donna Williams, Tito Mukhopadhyay and Wendy Lawson. Roth makes the point that "poetry, with its dependence on intensely abstract, symbolic, and free-flowing forms of expression" (p. 161) might be particularly suited to the autistic cognitive style.

Many features of Asperger syndrome enhance creativity, but the ability to focus deeply on a topic and to take endless pains is characteristic. Hans Asperger [24] emphasized the intensity with which special interests are pursued already in his first lecture about children with "autistic psychopathology". It appears that these unique qualities of concentration and also perception as discussed in subsequent paragraphs in individuals with ASD may give rise to extraordinary creative abilities. Exceptionally gifted people like for example the animal scientist and author Temple Grandin [25] declares that her autism, as manifested in her acute visual/spatial mind and in her powers of concentration is what has made her success possible (p.188). People with Asperger syndrome live very much in their intellects, and certain forms of creativity benefit greatly from this [26]. Apart from good concrete intelligence additional characteristics of a gifted person with ASD include, ability to disregard social conventions, unconcern about the opinions of others and a sometimes-childlike naivety and inquisitiveness.

According Nancy Andreasen [27], who made a significant contribution to research on creativity, the personality traits that characterize creative individuals include "openness to experience, adventuresomeness, rebelliousness, individualism, ... persistence, curiosity, simplicity, ... the ability to see things in a different and novel way, indifference to social conventions, dislike of externally imposed rules, driven by own set of rules derived from within and a childlike manner" (p.30-32). Not surprisingly, the above two descriptions are strikingly similar.

3. Cognitive processes involved in creativity

Creativity is a multidimensional construct and cognitive neuroscience is only beginning to understand the many cognitive components involved in creative thinking including the neural substrates underlying these processes [for a review see 28]. Theories of creativity in general suggest that creativity is linked to attentional capacity [29] and associative or divergent thinking processes [30]. Mendelsohn [31] emphasised the specific role of "defocused" attention or a widened attentional ability in highly creative individuals, which is in contrast with the extremely narrow focus of attention ascribed to individuals with autism [e.g. 32]. Likewise, divergent thinking, which involves the production of a variety of responses [33] and assumes to depend on extensively connected neural networks also conflicts with the well reported neural underconnectivity and enhanced local networks found in autism. As pointed out by Nettle [34] "different domains of creativity require different cognitive profiles, with poetry and art associated with divergent thinking, schizophrenia and affective disorder, and mathematics associated with convergent thinking and autism" (p.1). It appears that other concepts of information processing need to be considered when attempting to elucidate the specific and unique mechanisms underlying autistic creativity. In the words of Allan Snyder [35] "The fact that genius might fall within the autistic spectrum challenges our deepest notions of creativity. Are there radically different routes to creativity: normal and autistic?" (p. 1403).

The main current interpretation of special gifts and savant skills associated with autism include cognitive and psychological theories as well as various other models.

4. Savant syndrome and creativity

According to Treffert [36]: "Savant syndrome is a rare, but extraordinary condition in which persons with serious mental disabilities, including autistic disorder, have some 'island of genius' which stands in marked, incongruous contrast to overall handicap" (p.1351). Savant skills are found more commonly in ASD than in any other group [37] and are generally attributed to low-functioning autism but can also occur in individuals with normal and very high intelligence.

Theories put forward to explain savant skills strongly suggest a relationship with repetitive, obsessional and restricted behaviour [38]. Savants generally exhibit circumscribed interests usually within their skill area [39], which leads to considerable rehearsal, practice and training. Savant skills are also strongly associated with rote memory [40]. Pring [41] in her analysis of memory characteristics in savants argued against the rote memory explanation and instead proposed the existence of complex long-term memory structures in savants. In general, memory is considered an essential cognitive component of savant skills. In addition, researchers have suggested a role for 'implicit' or unintentional, learning in savant skill development [42,43]. Results of neuropsychological examinations of a calendar-calculating savant indicated that good memory, superior mental calculation and knowledge of calendar are the underlying elements for this specific talent [44]. Taken together, the classical portrait of the autistic savant is largely imitative and not very creative and some writers [e.g. 45] argued that true creativity is missing in savants "there are no savant geniuses about.... Their mental limitations disallow and preclude an awareness of innovative developments" (p. 177). In contrast, other theorists [46,47] believe that savants, particularly those with Asperger syndrome with above average intelligence levels [48] can be extremely creative. Mottron et al [49] write that "Savant performance cannot be reduced to uniquely efficient rote memory skills .... and encompasses not only the ability for strict recall, requiring pattern completion, but also the ability to produce creative, new material within the constraints of a previously integrated structure" (p.1388).

Various pathological conditions such as frontotemporal dementia, dominant-hemisphere strokes, head injuries and infections may also result in the emergence of savant like abilities [e.g. 50]. Of particular interest is the fact that individuals with these diverse types of disorders and emerging savant skills also develop cognitive features and behavioural traits, which are characteristic of autism [51].

5. Cognitive and psychological theories and explanations underlying special gifts and talents and savant skills in ASD

The development of special gifts and talents in ASD has been associated in general with the ability to process local information. These abilities include detail-focused cognitive style (weak coherence) [52], enhanced perceptual functioning [53], an accentuated capacity for systemizing [54], privileged access to low-level perceptual processes [55] and various other psychological and physiological states.

5.1. Weak central coherence

A different cognitive style, the weak central coherence theory (WCC) proposed by Uta Frith [56] and Frith and Happé [57] has been suggested as an explanation for certain special abilities found in ASD. This exceptional part-based processing style is demonstrated in the superior ability individuals with ASD show on tasks such as block design and embedded figures resulting from deficits in integration processes that serve to draw information together as a meaningful whole [see 58]. According to Frith [59], the WCC particularly addresses the special gifts and talents and acute perceptual abilities in autism (e.g. hypersensitivity, visual and auditory abilities) and can explain the achievements of individuals with ASD syndrome in art, science, music, and many other areas. Local coherence, which is defined by close attention to mechanical or physical patterns, is exemplified in the work of Temple Grandin [60]. Atypical attentional mechanisms and abnormal neural connectivity have been suggested as possible cognitive and neural mechanisms underlying WCC.

5.2. Enhanced perceptual functioning

Also located at the level of perception is the model proposed by Mottron and Burack [61] and Mottron et al [62] which are based on enhanced perceptual functioning (EPF) suggesting that people with autism have an overdevelopment of low-level perceptual abilities at the expense of high-level processing mechanisms. This theory provides a convincing account of special abilities in ASD such as peaks of ability in visual and auditory modalities and also indicates that a variety of cognitive processes are required for the development of savant abilities. For example, Mottron et al [63] propose that enhanced detection of patterns, including similarity within and among patterns is contributing to creativity evident in savants. As far as neural correlates for their theory is concerned the authors suggest the notion of brain plasticity and an overfunctioning of brain regions involved in perception in autism [64].

EPF and WCC are similar in emphasizing detail focused processing bias and superior local processing. Superiority in local coherence may be specific to autistic creativity and as argued by Mills [65] "produces an imaginative faculty defined by close attention to mechanical or physical patterns not psychological or social rules" (p.126).

5.3. Systemizing theory

This above interpretation appears to be in line with the "systemizing theory" put forward by Baron-Cohen et al. [66] which emphasises the superior ability in recognizing repeating patterns in stimuli (e.g. numerical, spatial, mechanical, auditory systemizing). The "systemizing theory", in contrast to the WCC model, predicts that individuals with ASD have a strong central coherence as indicated by their excellent skills in integrating information in areas such as astronomy and physics. This ability, however, does not apply to non-systemizable fields such as fiction. Similar to the WCC the systemizing model also posits excellent attention to detail in perception and memory. Baron-Cohen et al [67] further suggest that this excellent attention to detail is a consequence of sensory hypersensitivity found in individuals with ASD. Belmonte et al [68] posited that local overconnectivity in the posterior sensory parts of the cortex is responsible for the sensory 'magnification' in ASD.

5.4. Low level information processing

The work of Synder et al. [69] also provides an understanding of certain forms of creativity. According to Snyder and Mitchell [70] outstanding savant skills might be accomplished by accessing early stages of information processing. Their controversial model predicts the possibility of accessing non-conscious information by artificially disinhibiting the inhibiting networks associated with concept formation, using transcranial magnetic brain stimulation (TMS). By means of this method Snyder et al. [71] propose that this process will open "the door for restoration of perfect pitch, for recalling detail... and even enhancing creativity". A recent EEG study [72] attributing increased visual detail perception in autism to neural abnormalities related to low-level visual processing potentially supports this theory.

Snyders's theory [73] furthermore suggests the possibility that savant skills may be latent in everyone, but a "form of cortical disinhibition or atypical hemispheric imbalance" is required in order to access them (p. 1399). In support for his theory Snyder quotes the emergence of savant skills in individuals without any previous history for talents due to a variety of illnesses.

Snyder's model explains many of the talents and characteristics associated with Asperger geniuses including their childlike view of the world and lack of preconceptions, which is beneficial for developing new and original theories and perspectives. For example, Ludwig Wittgenstein, who had Asperger syndrome did spend little time reading other philosophers and felt most of them were wrong anyhow. He didn't want to "cloud his mind with false theories" [74].

5.5. Primary process thought and disinhibition syndrome, reduced self-awareness – 'Flow'

Theories of creativity [75, 76] also highlight the importance of primary process thought as found in dreaming, free association and psychosis in creative processes. Einstein suggested that creative scientists are the ones with "access to their dreams. Occasionally, a dream will actually provide the solution to a problem", as cited by Gregory [77] (p.226). Many mathematicians are intuitive thinkers and rely on the unconscious mind to a large extent, like for example the genius mathematician Poincarė [78]. Freudian theory holds that primary processes or primitive thinking which creative persons have more access to are based on their weak defence mechanisms of repression. Individuals with Asperger syndrome have very weak defence mechanisms thus allowing them access to early childhood memories [79].

Low levels of repression or inhibition are associated with creativity and a number of theorists [80, 81] have suggested that creativity is "a disinhibition syndrome", i.e. highly creative individuals lack cognitive inhibition. Neural correlates of cognitive disinhibition are the frontal lobes and research indicates that creative individuals show less frontal-lobe activity during verbal association tasks [82]. Deficits in inhibition have been documented in autism [83] as well as in Attention Deficit Hyperactivity Disorder (ADHD) [84] a neurodevelopmental disorder that is associated with increased creativity.

Also relevant in this context maybe the concept of "flow" proposed by the psychologist Csíkszentmihályi [85]. The notion of "flow" indicates a familiar state of reduced self-awareness where temporal concerns (time, food, ego-self, etc) are ignored during periods where the individual is fully immersed in a task or process. According to Csíkszentmihályi "flow" is characterised by a feeling of great absorption, engagement and fulfilment and thought to be inherently reinforcing and rewarding [86]. As alerted to in the chapter "Atypical Sense of Self in Autism Spectrum Disorders: A Neuro-cognitive Perspective" (this book) [87] diminished self-awareness which is a characteristic of individuals with ASD and associated with right hemisphere dysfunction might be advantageous in the development of special talents in ASD as quoted by Happé and Vital [88] (p.1373).

To conclude, although no single theory can explain the cognitive mechanisms underlying savant skill development, prodigious memory, atypical perception and excellent attention to detail are fundamentally associated with savant like talents in individual with ASD.

6. Neural basis of creativity in non-clinical populations

The study of the neural basis of creativity is an area greatly neglected by scientific research and despite methodological difficulties associated with investigating creativity any account of creativity must include explanations about the neural correlates of creativity [89].

Neuroscientific approaches aiming to determine the physiological basis of creative thought, are assuming that creativity is a measurable trait. Creativity can be interpreted as physiological changes that are required for creative problem solving focussing on EEG measures of cortical activation [90]. Theories of creativity in general postulate that low levels of cortical activation contribute to creative inspiration. Imaging data [91] suggest that great creativity not only requires a high level of specialized knowledge (stored in temporal and parietal lobes) and divergent thinking (mediated by the frontal lobes) but also co-activation and communication between areas of the brain that normally do not show strong connections. Highly creative individuals also possess the ability to modulate neurotransmitters [92, 93] such as the norepinephrine system (located in the frontal lobes), indicated by a reduction of cerebral levels of norepinephrine during creative periods. Support for the role of frontal areas in a fluid analogy-making task comes from an fMRI study [94] indicating bilateral neural activations. A study measuring differences in cerebral blood flow between highly creative individuals and controls during a verbal task of creative thinking [95] implicated a neural network consisting of right and left fronto-temporal, parietal, and cerebellar regions in highly creative performances. These areas are involved in cognition, emotion, working memory and response to novelty.

7. Neural basis of creativity in ASD

We are not aware of any studies investigating directly the neural basis of creativity in autism apart from studies exploring savant skills in autism. Some of these support the Left Hemisphere (LH) dysfunction/ and Right Hemisphere (RH) compensation theory [e.g. 96] as indicated by hemispheric asymmetry. Research evidence of neuroanatomical abnormalities including atypical minicolumnar organization in ASD [97,98] as well as neural hypotheses about abnormal connectivity [e.g. 99] support this theory.

7.1. Hemispheric asymmetry

Cerebral asymmetry refers to the lack of structural symmetry in left and right hemispheres in humans. Atypical cerebral asymmetry, a deviation from the normal pattern of cerebral asymmetry has been associated with special cognitive talents [100] and creativity [101] as cited by Smalley et al. [102]. For example, the capability for making distal or global verbal associations is one factor contributing to creativity and according to Brugger and Graves [103] the basis for this type of verbal creativity is "cerebral laterality in which an individual has a relative weakening of left hemisphere dominance and strengthening of availability of right hemisphere processing" [104] p. 138.

Atypical cerebral asymmetry has been associated with autism, dyslexia and ADHD [105], neurodevelopmental disorders considered to share regions of linkage overlap [106]. In addition, creativity in psychiatric populations is often associated with atypical cerebral asymmetry [107] and a RH "bias" [108].

Research evidence for atypical cerebral asymmetry in autism (e.g. increased size of some RH cortical structures) and reversed lateralization of language has been well documented [e.g. 109]. An imaging study by Herbert et al [110] found a "sizeable right-asymmetry increase" in subjects with autism. Individuals with autism had twice as much right-as left-asymmetrical cortex than the control sample. This finding was interpreted as a consequence of early abnormal brain growth abnormalities. According to the hypothesis put forward by Geschwind and Galaburda [111] the immaturity of the LH in utero makes it more susceptible to damage, which could result in a compensatory overdevelopment of the RH caused by neural migration and thus resulting in an anomalous RH-dominance. As the RH develops earlier than the LH, accelerated early brain development in autism may lead to anomalous lateralization of cognitive functions as suggested by Herbert et al [112].

7.2. Right hemisphere processing and creativity

Savant skills are linked to the RH [113], which is dominant for attention, visuospatial and emotional function. Various authors [114-115] have suggested that autistic savants have atypical LH dysfunction with RH compensation. Based on research evidence including imaging studies Treffert [116] speculated that "one mechanism in some savants, whether congenital or acquired is left brain dysfunction with right brain compensation." The notion of "paradoxical functional facilitation" as described by Kapur [117] denotes loss of function in one damaged brain area and enhanced function of another area, which as emphasized by Treffert is "central to explaining savant syndrome" (p.1356).

RH skills can be characterized as non-symbolic, artistic, concrete and directly perceived in contrast to LH skills that are more sequential, logical, and symbolic. For example musical, artistic, visual or spatial abilities (mathematics) are primarily RH skills.

The association between RH and creativity is based on research evidence demonstrating that the RH is more involved in production of mental images than the LH, perception and production of music, e.g. the right inferior frontal gyrus is known to be involved in musical pitch encoding and melodic pitch memory [118]. EEG studies show that highly creative individuals show more right than left-hemisphere activation during experimental studies [119], indicating that during the creative process creative individuals rely more on the RH. Lesion studies as well as unimpaired population studies have demonstrated that the RH is superior to the LH at noticing anomalies in objects [120]. Individuals with autism are well known for detecting even the smallest changes in the environment.

In sum, several lines of evidence suggest that atypical cerebral asymmetry which is a highly heritable trait [121] is associated with autism and linked to certain aspects of creativity. It is also likely that some of the structural brain abnormalities evidenced in autism are related to the special cognitive functioning that encourages great creativity. Neurological brain differences have been reported in the literature on creativity [122].

7.3. Neuroanatomical abnormalities in autism

Converging neuroscientific evidence has suggested that the neuropathology of ASD is widely distributed, involving impaired connectivity throughout the brain. Neuroanatomical abnormalities in autism include increase in cortical thickness [123], and increase in head and brain size [124]. Accelerated growth in brain size in early childhood in autism has been documented by a range of studies [125], which may be consistent with the asymmetric cerebral lateralization in autism as discussed above. The increased brain volumes in autism are believed to be the result of insufficient or abnormal prenatal pruning, which together with genetic factors are most likely to underlie these growth abnormalities [126]. In addition, there is evidence of higher birth weight [127] and faster body growth [128] as well as increased levels of growth hormones [129] in autism. These altered brain growth rates are considered to have a strong influence on patterns of brain connectivity and cerebral lateralization [130, 131] and differential cognitive functioning. For example, the increased hippocampus size in autism [132] may be associated with enhanced visual-spatial, mathematical and mechanistic processing in autism as well as savant abilities such as calculation and memory. Imaging data of a reduced size of corpus callosum in autism [133] is consistent with the reduced interhemispheric brain connectivity reported in autistic individuals [134]. Neural underconnectivity [e.g. 135] provides support for the weak "central coherence theory" which postulates enhanced local and decreased global information processing in autism. Research on patterns of cortical connectivity also indicates that a specific minicolumnar phenotype found in autism may be beneficial for information processing and/or focused attention and may also offer an explanation for the savant abilities autism [136, 137].

To conclude, although neural mechanisms underlying savant skill and development are not well established, associating creativity with hemisphere lateralization and anatomical abnormalities in autism is supported by empirical evidence and also has some explanatory potential. Additional areas to explore are genetic factors and creativity found in other pathological conditions.

8. Nature versus nurture

Is great creativity a fortunate combination of specific traits, or do "creativity genes" exist? As speculated by Smalley et al [138] "genes that increase one's risk for certain psychiatric or learning disorders may also be 'enhancer' genes for creativity (and intuition)" (p.82). According to Gardner [139] it is extremely unlikely that there is such a thing as a "poetry gene or a music gene" since complex human behaviours typically have a "polygenic basis" (p. 175). Without doubt ASD have a polygenic basis and genetic factors not only contribute to specific skills but also to traits such as persistence, the capacity for concentration for extended periods, and curiosity about certain types of stimulation. Lykken et al [140] describe the concept of *emergenesis*, an extreme form of epitasis, in which a unique combination of genes may lead to qualitative shifts in capacity or ability that may apply to extremely gifted individuals with ASD.

The relationship between inherited talent and/or extensive practice is a very contentious aspect of superior ability in specific skills. The view propounded by Howe [141] emphasizing the overwhelming role of practice in the acquirement of special skills, is largely rejected by a majority of theorists who argue for the role of innate talent [142-144]. Special talents are essentially innate in predisposing to cognitive or physical qualities and are the key to understanding geniuses from Einstein to Mozart [145]. For example, research evidence from twin data [146] suggests a genetic basis for detail-focused cognitive style predisposing to talent in ASD. It is configuration of genes and variations in genetic inputs that are critical to the success in persons of great creativity. It is our belief that there are significant genetic underpinnings to creativity of genius proportions, which of course could not be expressed without environmental factors.

9. Novelty, ADHD and creativity

The majority of theoretical conceptions of creativity agree that the main component of creativity is its novelty, uniqueness or unusualness that undoubtedly applies to the creativity displayed by gifted individuals with ASD. Novelty or sensation seeking behaviour is also strongly associated with ADHD. A significant degree of comorbidity between autism and ADHD has been documented [e.g. 147] in the literature. Although reported to have poor attention and concentration and being poor academic performers individuals with ADHD have a capacity to hyperfocus, which allows them to produce great works of art. For example the poetry of Lord Byron, who had ADHD [148] is an example for a work of genius in this area. As pointed out above, both autism and ADHD are associated with atypical cerebral asymmetry which is a highly heritable and complex phenotype linked to creativity and sharing regions of linkage overlap [149,150].

10. Psychopathology

There is a very close relationship between creativity (especially in literature and arts) and psychopathology, particularly mood disorder [151, 152]. An association of biochemical factors in psychosis and creativity has been suggested by Folley et al [153] indicating the noradrenergic system. This model also provides possible links between attention, divergent thinking, and arousal based on mechanisms that interact with structural and neurochemical systems of the brain and has the potential to explain the novelty seeking behaviour implicated in ADHD but may have less explanatory power as far as autism is concerned. According to Sternberg and Lubart [154] creativity and novelty must be coupled with appropriateness for something to be considered creative. Although schizotypal thought most likely leads to an increase in novel ideas, they may not always be appropriate.

In contrast, the nature of creativity displayed by individuals with ASD is associated with the distinctiveness of the autistic brain and its unique neural connectivity. In this context Temple Grandin [155] has stated, "it is likely that genius is an abnormality" (p178-179). However, she also believes that autistic intelligence is necessary in order to add diversity and creativity to the world: "It is possible that persons with bits of these traits are more creative, are possibly even geniuses...If science eliminated these genes, maybe the whole world would be taken over by accountants" (p.124).

11. Conclusion

The results of our evaluation suggest that many features of ASD are advantageous for great creativity. Creativity is an extremely complex and multifaceted construct and no cognitive theory or model of brain function has so far been able to fully account for it. We suggest that the distinctive gifts of perception, attention, memory and information processing combined with personality attributes can give rise to the extraordinary creativity seen in some individuals with ASD. It is our view that progress in elucidating the neural basis of autism may hold promises for a better understanding of autistic creativity and creativity in general. Autism Spectrum Disorders are mainly portrayed as negative phenomena, as a curse, but if they were an integral part of the mindset of highly creative individuals such as Einstein and Darwin who possessed autistic traits they could be regarded in some aspects as a gift [156].

Author details

Viktoria Lyons* and Michael Fitzgerald

*Address all correspondence to: viktorialyons@yahoo.co.uk

Trinity College Dublin, Ireland

References

[1] Griffiths TD. Scientific Commentary. Capturing Creativity. Brain 2008;131: 6-7.

[2] Baird G, Cox A, Charman, T, Baron-Cohen S. et al. A Screening Instrument for Autism at 18 Months of Age: A Six-Year Follow-up Study. Journal of the American Academy of Child and Adolescent Psychiatry 2000; 39: 694-702.

[3] Happé F. Communicative Competence and Theory of Mind in Autism: A Test of Relevance Theory. Cognition 1993;48: 101-119.

[4] Bruner J, Feldman C. Theories of Mind and the Problem of Autism. In: Baron-Cohen S, Tager-Flusberg H, Cohen DJ. (eds) Understanding Other Minds: Perspectives from Autism. Oxford: Oxford University Press; 1993. p 267-291.

[5] Baron-Cohen S. Theory of Mind and Autism: a Review. Special Issue of The International Review of Mental Retardation 2001; 23: 169.

[6] Craig J, Baron-Cohen S. Creativity and Imagination in Autism and Asperger Syndrome. Journal of Autism and Developmental Disorders 1999;29: 319-326

[7] Fitzgerald M. Autism and Creativity: Is there a link between autism in men and exceptional ability? New York: Brunner Routledge; 2004.

[8] Fitzgerald M. The Genesis of Artistic Creativity. London: Jessica Kingsley; 2005.

[9] Fitzgerald M, James I. The Mind of the Mathematician. Baltimore: John Hopkins Press; 2007.

[10] Sacks O. An Anthropologist on Mars: Seven Paradoxical Tales. New York: Knopf; 1995.

[11] Treffert DA. The savant syndrome: an extraordinary condition. A synopsis: past, present, future. In: Happé F, Frith U. (eds.) Autism and talent. Philosophical transactions of The Royal Society 2009; vol. 364 (1522) p1351-1358.

[12] Mottron L, Dawson M, Soulières I. Enhanced perception in savant syndrome: patterns, structure and creativity. In: Happé F, Frith U. (eds.) Autism and talent. Philosophical transactions of The Royal Society 2009; vol. 364 (1522) p1385-1392.

[13] Asperger H. Die autistischen Psychopathen im Kindesalter. Archiv fuer Psychiatrie und Nervenkrankheiten 1944;11: 76-136.

[14] Jay E. Problem finding: understanding its nature and mechanism. Qualifying paper, Harvard Graduate School of Education, Cambridge, M.A.; 1989.

[15] Lincoln AJ, Allen MH, Kilman A. The assessment and interpretation of intellectual abilities in people with Autism. In: Schopler E, Mesibov GB (eds.). Learning and cognition in autism. New York: Plenum Press; 1995. p89-117.

[16] Dawson M, Soulieres I, Gernsbacher MA, Mottron L. The level and nature of autistic intelligence. Psychological Science 2007;18: 657-662.

[17] Scheuffgen K, Happé F, Anderson M, Frith U. High 'intelligence,' low 'IQ' Speed of processing and measured IQ in children with autism. Developmental Psychopathology 2000;12: 83-90.

[18] Sternberg RJ, O'Hara LA. Intelligence and Creativity. In: Sternberg RJ. (ed.) Handbook of Intelligence. Cambridge: Cambridge University Press; 2000.

[19] Guilford JP. Creativity. American Psychologist 1950;5: 444-454.

[20] Lubart T. In Search of Creative Intelligence. In: Sternberg J, Lautrey J, Lubart TI (eds.) Models of intelligence: international perspectives. Washington: APA; 2004.

[21] Heilman KM, Nadeau SE, Beversdorf DO. Creative Innovation: Possible Brain Mechanism. Neurocase 2003;9: 369-379.

[22] Gardner H. Frames of mind: The theory of multiple intelligences. New York: Basic; 1983.

[23] Roth I. Imagination and the Awareness of Self in Autistic Spectrum Poets. In: Osteen M. (ed.) Autism and Representation. New York: Routledge; 2008.

[24] Asperger H. Das psychisch abnorme Kind. Wiener Klinische Wochenzeitschrift 1938;49: 1314-1317.

[25] Grandin, T. Thinking in Pictures: and Other Reports from my Life with Autism. New York: Doubleday; 1995.

[26] Fitzgerald & James, 2007.

[27] Andreasen NC. The Creating Brain. The Neuroscience of Genius. New York: Dana Press; 2005.

[28] Abraham A, Windmann S. Creative cognition: The diverse operations and the prospect of applying a cognitive neuroscience perspective. Methods 2007; 22: 38-8.

[29] Mendelsohn GA. Associative and attentional processes in creative performance. Journal of Personality 1976;44: 341-369.

[30] Guilford JP. The nature of human intelligence. New York: McGraw-Hill; 1967.

[31] Mendelsohn 1976.

[32] Townsend J, Courchesne E. Parietal damage and narrow 'spotlight' spatial attention. Journal of Cognitive Neuroscience 1994;6: 220-232.

[33] Torrance EP. The Torrance Tests of Creative Thinking: Technical-norms manual. Bensenville, IL: Scholastic Testing Service; 1974.

[34] Nettle D. Schizotypy and mental health amongst poets, visual artists, and mathematicians. Journal of Research in Personality 2006;40: 876-890.

[35] Snyder A. Explaining and inducing savant skills: privileged access to lower level, less-processed information. In: Happé F, Frith U. (eds.) Autism and talent. Philosophical transactions of The Royal Society 2009; vol. 364 (1522) p1399-1406.

[36] Treffert 2009.

[37] Howlin P, Goode S, Hutton J, Rutter M. Savant skills in autism: psychometric approaches and parental reports. In: Happé F, Frith U. (eds.) Autism and talent. Philosophical transactions of The Royal Society 2009; vol. 364 (1522) p1369-1368.

[38] O'Connor N, Hermelin B. Talents and preoccupations in idiot-savants. Psychological Medicine 1991;21: 959-964.

[39] O'Connor & Hermelin, 1991.

[40] Hill AL. Savants: Mentally retarded individuals with special skills. In Ellis N. (ed.) International review of research in mental retardation. New York: Academic Press; 1978. (9) p277-298.

[41] Pring L. Memory characteristics in individuals with savant skills. In: Boucher J, Bowler D. (eds.) Memory in Autism. Cambridge: Cambridge University Press; 2008.

[42] Treffert D. Extraordinary people: understanding 'idiot savants'. New York: Harper and Row; 1989.

[43] Hermelin B. Bright splinters of the mind: a personal story of research with autistic savants. London: Jessica Kingsley Press; 2001.

[44] Wallace GL, Happé F, Giedd JN. A case study of a multiply talented savant with an autism spectrum disorder: neuropsychological functioning and brain morphometry.

In: Happé F, Frith U. (eds.) Autism and talent. Philosophical transactions of The Royal Society 2009; vol. 364 (1522) p1425-1432.

[45] Hermelin 2001.

[46] Treffert 2009.

[47] Mottron, Dawson & Soulières 2009.

[48] Fitzgerald 2005.

[49] Mottron, Dawson & Soulières 2009.

[50] Seeley WW, Matthews BR, Crawford RK, Gorno-Tempini ML, Foti D, Mackenzie IR, Miller BL. Unravelling Boléro: progressive aphasia, transmodal creativity and the right posterior neocortex. Brain 2008;131: 39-49.

[51] Heaton P. Wallace GL. Annotation: The savant syndrome. Journal of Child Psychology and Psychiatry 2004;45: 899-911.

[52] Frith U, Happė F. Autism: beyond "theory of mind". Cognition 1994;50: 115-132.

[53] Mottron, Dawson & Soulières 2009.

[54] Baron-Cohen S, Ashwin E, Ashwin C, Tavassoli T, Chakrabarti B. Talent in autism: hyper-systemizing, hyper-attention to detail and sensory hypersensitivity. In: Happé F, Frith U. (eds.) Autism and talent. Philosophical transactions of The Royal Society 2009; vol. 364 (1522) p1377-1384.

[55] Snyder AW, Mitchell DJ. Is integer arithmetic fundamental to mental processing? the mind's secret arithmetic. London: Proceedings of the Royal Society 1999;266: 587-592.

[56] Frith U. Autism: Explaining the Enigma. Oxford: Blackwell; 1989.

[57] Frith & Happė 1994.

[58] Happé F, Frith U. The Weak Coherence Account: detail-focused Cognitive style in Autism Spectrum Disorders. Journal of Autism and Developmental Disorders 2006;36: 5-25.

[59] Frith, U. (2004). Emanuel Miller lecture: Confusions and controversies about Asperger Syndrome. Journal of Child Psychology and Psychiatry 2004;45: 672-686, p. 680.

[60] Grandin 1995.

[61] Mottron L, Burack JA. Enhanced perceptual functioning in the development of autism. In: Burack JA, Charman T, Yirmiya N, Zelazo PR. (eds.) The development of autism: Perspectives from theory and research. New Jersey: Lawrence Erlbaum; 2001.

[62] Mottron L, Dawson M, Soulières I, Hubert B, Burack J. Enhanced Perceptual functioning in Autism: An Update, and eight Principles of Autistic Perception. Journal of Autism and Developmental Disorders 2006;3: 27-43.

[63] Mottron, Dawson & Soulières 2009.

[64] Mottron & Burack 2001.

[65] Mills B. Autism and the Imagination. In: Osteen M. (ed.) Autism and Representation. New York: Routledge; 2008.

[66] Baron-Cohen S, Richler J, Bisarya D, Gurunathan N, Wheelwright S. The systemizing quotient: an investigation of adults with Asperger syndrome or high-functioning autism and normal sex differences. In: Frith U, Hill E. (eds.) Autism: Mind and Brain. Oxford: Oxford University Press; 2004. p161-186.

[67] Baron-Cohen et al. 2009.

[68] Belmonte MK, Allen G, Beckel-Mitchener A, Boulanger LM, Carper RA, Webb SJ. Autism and abnormal development of brain connectivity. Journal of Neuroscience 2004;24: 9228-31.

[69] Snyder AW, Bossomaier T, Mitchell DJ. Concept Formation: Object Attributes Dynamically Inhibited from Conscious Awareness. Journal of Integrative Neuroscience 2004;(3) 1: 31–46.

[70] Snyder & Mitchell 1999.

[71] Snyder et al 2004.

[72] Vandenbroucke MWG, Scholte HS, van Engeland H, Lamme VAF, Kemner C. A neural substrate for atypical low-level visual processing in autism spectrum disorder. Brain 2008, 131(4): 1013-1024.

[73] Snyder 2009.

[74] Fitzgerald 2004.

[75] Freud S. Creative writers and daydreaming. In: Strachey J. (ed. & trans.) Standard edition of the complete psychological works of Sigmund Freud. London: Hogarth Press; 1959. (9) p141-153.

[76] Kris E. Psychoanalytic explorations in art. New York: International Universities Press; 1952.

[77] Gregory FL. The Oxford Companion to the Mind. Oxford: Oxford University Press; 2004.

[78] Fitzgerald & James, 2005.

[79] Lyons V, Fitzgerald, M. Early Memory and Autism. Letter to the Editor. Journal of Autism and Developmental Disorders 2005;35: 683.

[80] Eysenck H. Genius: The natural history of creativity. Cambridge: Cambridge University Press; 1995.

[81] Martindale C. Personality, situation, and creativity. In: Glover JA, Running RR, Reynolds CR (eds.) Handbook of creativity. New York: Plenum; 1989. p211-228.

[82] Hudspith S. The neurological correlates of creative thought. Unpublished PhD. Dissertation, University of Southern California, Los Angeles, CA; 1985.

[83] Johnson KA, Robertson IH, Kelly SP. et al. Dissociation in performance of children with ADHD and high-functioning autism on a task of sustained attention. Neuropsychologia 2007;45: 2234-2245.

[84] Ozonoff, S. Components of executive function in autism and other disorders. In: Russell J. (ed.) Autism as an Executive Disorder. Oxford: Oxford University Press; 1997.

[85] Csíkszentmihályi M. Flow: the psychology of optimal experience. Ney York: Harper and Row; 1990.

[86] Csíkszentmihályi M, Lefevre J. Optimal experience in work and leisure. Journal of Personal and Social Psychology 1989;56: 815-822.

[87] Lyons V, Fitzgerald M. Atypical Sense of Self in Autism Spectrum Disorders: A Neuro-cognitive Perspective. In: ....

[88] Happé F, Vital P. What aspects of autism predispose to talent? In: Happé F, Frith U. (eds.) Autism and talent. Philosophical transactions of The Royal Society 2009; vol. 364 (1522): p1369-1376.

[89] Zeki S. Essays on science and society. Artistic creativity and the brain. Science 2001;293: 51-2.

[90] Martindale C. Creative imagination and neural activity. In: Kunzendorf R, Sheikh A. (eds.) Psychophysiology of mental imagery: Theory, research, and application. Amityville, NY: Baywood; 1990. p89-108.

[91] Heilman, Nadeau & Beversdorf, 2003.

[92] Beversdorf DQ, Hughes JD, Steinberg BA, Lewis LD, Heilman KM. Noradrenergic modulation of cognitive flexibility in problem solving. Neuroreport 1999;10: 2763-7.

[93] Folley BS, Doop ML, Park S. Psychoses and creativity: is the missing link a biological mechanism related to phospholipids turnover? Prostaglandins, Leukotrienes and Essential Fatty Acids 2003;69: 467-476.

[94] Gaeke JG, Hansen PC. Neural correlates of intelligence as revealed by fMRI of fluid analogies. Neuroimage 2005;26: 555-64.

[95] Chavez-Eakle RA, Graff-Guerrero A, Garcia-Reyna JC, Vaugier V, Cruz-Fuentes D. Cerebral blood flow associated with creative performance: a comparative study. Neuroimage 2007;38: 519-28.

[96] Rimland B. Infantile Autism: the Syndrome and its implications for a neural theory of behavior. New York: Appleton-Century-Crofts; 1978.

[97] Casanova MF, Switala AE, Trippe J, Fitzgerald M. Comparative minicolumnar morphometry of three distinguished scientists. Autism, The International Journal of Research and Practice 2007;11: 55-569.

[98] Casanova M, Trippe J. Radial cytoarchitecture and patterns of cortical connectivity in autism. In: Happé F, Frith U. (eds.) Autism and talent. Philosophical transactions of The Royal Society 2009; vol. 364 (1522) p1433-1436.

[99] Belmonte et al 2004.

[100] Geschwind N, Miller BL. Molecular approaches to cerebral laterality: development and neurodegeneration. American Journal of Medical Genetics 2001;101: 379-381.

[101] Brugger P, Graves R.E. Right hemispatial inattention and magical ideation. European Archive for Psychiatry Clinical Neuroscience 1997;247: 55-57.

[102] Smalley SL, Loo SK, Yang MH, Cantor RM. Toward Localizing Genes Underlying Cerebral Asymmetry and Mental Health. American Journal of Medical Genetics Part B (Neuropsychiatric Genetics) 2004;135B: 79-84.

[103] Brugger & Graves, 1997.

[104] Weinstein S, Graves RE. Are creativity and schizotypy products of a right hemisphere bias? Brain Cognition 2002;49: 138-151.

[105] Smalley et al 2004.

[106] Smalley SL, Kustanovich V, Minassian S, Stone JL, Ogdie MN. et al. Genetic linkage of attention-deficit/hyperactivity disorder on chromosome 16p13, in a region implicated in autism. American Journal Human Genetics 2002;71: 959-963.

[107] Overby LA III, Harris AE, Leek MR. Perceptual asymmetry in schizophrenia and affective disorder: Implications from a right hemisphere task. Neuropsychologia 1989;27: 861-870.

[108] Weinstein & Graves 2002.

[109] Bigler ED, Mortensen S, Neeley ES, Ozonoff S, Krasny, L, Johnson M, Lu J, Provencal SL, McMahon W, Lainhart, JE. Superior temporal gyrus, language function, and autism. Developmental Neuropsychology 2007;31: 217-38.

[110] Herbert MR, Ziegler DA, Deutsch CK, O'Brien LM, Kennedy DN, Filipek PA, Barkardjiev AI, Hodgson J, Takeoka M, Makris N, Caviness Jr VS. Brain asymmetries in autism and developmental language disorder: a nested whole-brain analysis. Brain 2005;28: 213-226.

[111] Geschwind N, Galaburda AM. Cerebral Lateralization: Biological Mechanisms, Associations, and Pathology. Cambridge: MIT Press; 1987.

[112] Herbert et al 2005.

[113] Treffert D. The idiot savant: a review of the syndrome. American Journal of Psychiatry 2000; 45: 563-572.

[114] Miller BL, Boone K, Cummings LR, Mishkin F. Emergence of artistic talent in frontotemporal dementia. Neurology 1998;51: 978-982.

[115] Sacks O. Musicophilia: tales of music and the brain. New York: Knopf Publishing Group; 2007.

[116] Treffert 2009.

[117] Kapur N. Paradoxical functional facilitation in brain-behaviour research: a critical review. Brain 1996;119 1775-1790.

[118] Hyde K, Zatorre R, GriffithsTD, Lerch JP, Peretz I. Morphometry of the amusic brain: A two-site study. Brain 2006;129:2562-70.

[119] Martindale C, Hines D, Mitchell L, Covello E. EEG alpha asymmetry and creativity. Personality and Individual Differences 1984;5: 77-86.

[120] Smith SD, Dixon MJ, Tays WJ, Bulman-Fleming MB. Anomaly detection in the right hemisphere: The influence of visuospatial factors. Brain Cognition 2004;55: 458-62.

[121] Geschwind DH, Miller BL, DeCarli C, Carmelli D. Heritability of lobar brain volumes in twins supports genetic models of cerebral laterality and handedness. Proceedings of the National Academy of Sciences USA 2002;99: 3176-3181

[122] Herrmann N. The creative brain. Lake Lure, N.C: Applied Creative Services; 1988.

[123] Hardan AY, Muddasani S, Vemulapalli M, Keshavan MS, Minshew NJ. An MRI study of increased cortical thickness in autism. American Journal of Psychiatry 2006;163: 1290-92.

[124] Dissanayake C, Bui QM, Huggins R, Loesch DZ. Growth in stature and head circumference in high-functioning autism and Asperger disorder during the first 3 years of life. Development and Psychopathology 2006;18: 381-93.

[125] Courchesne E, Pierce K. Brain overgrowth in autism during a critical time in development: Implications for frontal pyramidal neuron and interneuron development and connectivity. International Journal of Developmental Neuroscience 2005; 23: 153-70.

[126] Courchesne E. Brain development in autism: Early overgrowth followed by premature arrest of growth. Mental retardation and Developmental Disabilities. Research Reviews 2004;10 106-11.

[127] Mraz KD, Green J, Dumont-Mathieu T, Makin S, Fein D. Correlates of head circumference growth in infants later diagnosed with autism spectrum disorders. Journal of Child Neurology 2007;22: 700-13.

[128] Dissanayake et al 2006.

[129] Mills JL, Hediger ML, Molloy CA, et al. Elevated levels of growth-related hormones in autism and autism spectrum disorder. Clinical Endocrinology 2007;67: 230-37.

[130] Crespi B, Badcock C. Psychosis and autism as diametrical disorders of the social brain. Behavioral and Brain Sciences 2008;31: 284-320.

[131] Turner KC, Frost L, Linsenbardt D, McIlroy JR, Müller RA. Atypically diffuse functional connectivity between caudate nuclei and cerebral cortex. Behavioural and Brain Functions 2006;2 34.

[132] Schumann KC, Hamstra J, Goodlin-Jones BL, Lotspeich LJ, et al. The amygdala is enlarged in children but nor adolescents with autism; the hippocampus is enlarged at all ages. Journal of Neuroscience 2004; 25: 6392-6401.

[133] Egaas B, Courchesne E, Saitoh O. Reduced size of corpus callosum in autism. Archives of Neurology 1995; 52: 794-801.

[134] Belmonte et al 2004.

[135] Just MA, Cherkassky VL, Keller TA. Kana, RK, Minshew N. (Functional and Anatomical Cortical Underconnectivity in autism: Evidence from a fMRI Study of an Executive function task and Corpus Callosum Morphometry. Cerebral Cortex 2007;17: 951-961.

[136] Casanova et al 2007.

[137] Casanova et al 2009.

[138] Smalley et al 2004.

[139] Gardner H. Extraordinary Minds. New York: Basic Books; 1997.

[140] Lykken DT. The mechanism of emergenesis. Genes, Brain & Behavior 2006;5: 306-310.

[141] Howe MA. Genius Explained. Cambridge: Cambridge University Press; 1999.

[142] Happé F, Frith U. The beautiful otherness of the autistic mind. Introduction. appé F, Frith U. (eds.) Autism and talent. Philosophical transactions of The Royal Society 2009; vol. 364 (1522) p.1345-1350.

[143] Fitzgerald 2004.

[144] Fitzgerald 2005.

[145] Fitzgerald 2005.

[146] Happé &Vital 2009.

[147] Goldstein S. Schwebach AJ. A comorbidity of pervasive developmental disorder and Attention Deficit Hyperactivity Disorder: results of a retrospective chart review. Journal of Autism & Developmental Disorders 2004;34 (3): 329-339.

[148] Fitzgerald M. Did Lord Byron have Attention Deficit Hyperactivity Disorder? Journal of Medical Biography 2001;9: 31-33.

[149] Smalley et al 2002.

[150] Smalley et al 2004.

[151] Andreasen NC. Creativity and mental illness: prevalence rates in writers and their first-degree relatives. American Journal of Psychiatry 1987;144: 1288-1292.

[152] Andreasen NC 1987.

[153] Folley et al 2003.

[154] Sternberg RJ, Lubart TI. Defying the crowd: Cultivating creativity in a culture of conformity. New York: Free Press; 1995.

[155] Grandin 1995.

[156] Lyons V, Fitzgerald M. Asperger Syndrome. A Gift or a Curse? New York: Nova Science Publishers; 2005.

Chapter 9

Atypical Sense of Self in Autism Spectrum Disorders: A Neuro-Cognitive Perspective

Viktoria Lyons and Michael Fitzgerald

Additional information is available at the end of the chapter

1. Introduction

1.1. Self – Definitions and concepts

The concept of self is notoriously difficult to define and different notions and theories of the self have been proposed by a variety of disciplines all interpreting concepts of self and identity in various ways. We adopt the definition advanced by neuroscientists Kircher and David [1] who interpret the self as 'the commonly shared experience, that we know we are the same person across time, that we are the author of our thoughts/actions, and that we are distinct from the environment' (p.2). In cognitive neuroscience literature, operational definitions of the self are used which are measurable by experimental methods including self recognition, self and other differentiation, body awareness, awareness of other minds, awareness of self as expressed in language and important concepts such as autobiographical memory and self narrative. There is significant interest in the role of the self and possible abnormalities associated with the self, as causally implicated in autism. In this paper we review developmental perspectives of self and self-related functions with reference to their neuroanatomical basis and investigate the possible causes for atypical self-development in Autism Spectrum Disorders (ASD).

2. Review of studies investigating the self in ASD

The question whether individuals with ASD have a different sense of self than people without ASD, i.e. 'neurotypicals' has fascinated researchers and clinicians for decades. Kanner [2] in 1943 already noted self-deficits in the children he described, including their difficulties in maintaining a constant self-concept, and associated problems of adapting their fragile self-concept to changing environments. Asperger [3] (1974, p. 2026) refers to a disturbance and a weakness of the self in children with 'autistic psychopathy'. Psychoanalytic theories considered autism as a disorder of the self [4] based on the lack of ability in establishing stable internal representations of themselves and of others. The German psychiatrist Lutz [5] (1968) interpreted autism as a disturbance of self-consciousness, self-related activities and self-perception. Powell and Jordan [6] (1993) suggested that individuals with ASD lack an 'experiencing self' that provides a personal dimension for ongoing events. This is consistent with Frith's [7] suggestion of an 'absent self' in autism. Hobson [8] put forward a developmental account of the self in autism emphasising impaired interpersonal relatedness, 'intersubjectivity' and its far-reaching consequences for the development of the self. In a recent study investigating whether children with autism show abnormal self-other connectedness, Hobson and Meyer [9] found a failure in autism to identify with another person. These authors suggest that this process of identifying with others is crucial for a normal development of self-other relationship and the basis for understanding other minds.

3. Atypical development of self-related processes in ASD

There is general consensus among developmental theorists [e.g. 10,11] that early interpersonal communication is central to the establishment of the self in normal development. A large body of research literature indicates that early processes underlying self-other awareness are impaired or delayed in autism including gaze following, abnormal response to sound and deficits in attention [12], showing of objects, responding and orienting to own name [13], looking at other's faces [14], pretend play, protodeclarative pointing and gaze monitoring [15], empathy and imitation [16], joint-attention behaviour [17], affect and personal relatedness [18,19].

3.1. Self recognition and awareness

The ability to recognize one's own face in the mirror is considered a test for 'self-awareness'. Self-recognition as measured by mirror tests [20] in 18 months old children has been depicted as a developmental milestone in self-conception and described as the 'achievement of a cognitive self' [21]. Not only is self recognition essential for developing a concept of self, and self-other differentiation, it is also a prerequisite for later developing theory of mind abilities, as a stable self concept is the basis for being able to read the mental states of others. Research data on self-recognition reveals that autistic children's responses to their mirror images are qualitatively different from those of normal children [22]. Children with ASD have deficits of self-awareness as measured by a self-recognition test [23] they show little interest in their own mirror images and have been described as relatively 'face inexperienced' [24].

The prefrontal cortex, especially the Right Hemisphere (RH) plays a critical role in the recognition of one's own face [25] as evidenced by functional imaging studies. Face perception studies in individuals with ASD suggest abnormal functioning in the fusiform face area as well as amygdala, brain regions associated with the 'social brain' (e.g. 26,27] involving the RH.

3.2. Self/other differentiation

The ability to differentiate between self and other is also essential for the development of self-awareness, which appears to be impaired in autism. In particular, the recognition of a separate existence of other people seems to be delayed in children with autism [28,29]. Attentional abnormalities, such as 'tunnel vision', the tendency to think in a monotropic manner have been suggested by some as the cause of 'self-other problems' in ASD [30]. Donna Williams [31] interprets monoprocessing as the inability to process simultaneously information of oneself and others.

In neurotypicals the middle cingulate cortex and ventromedial prefrontal cortex are involved in self/other processing. In contrast, atypical neural responses have been reported in individuals with ASD. A recent fMRI study [32] investigating the attribution of behavioural outcomes to either oneself or others while playing an interactive trust game revealed a lack of brain activity in the cingulate cortex indicating diminished 'self responses' in individuals with ASD. However, 'other responses', attributing actions to other people were intact. Previous research data using trust games [33] had demonstrated that cingulate cortex activation is consistent with self-response patterns generated during interpersonal exchanges. Chiu et al. [34] interpreted their data in terms of a deficit in ASD in monitoring their own intentions in social interactions and thus contributing to impaired theory of mind abilities, lack of introspection and self-referential processing. Of particular interest is the fact that the 'impaired self-responses' in the ASD group correlated with their behavioural symptom severity, i.e. the lesser activity along cingulated cortex the more serious were their behavioural symptoms. Similar results have been reported by Lombardo et al. [35] also demonstrating atypical neural responses from the middle cingulate cortex during a self-referential processing task. This study also provided a link between these deficits and early social impairments in autism. In addition, these authors also demonstrated reduced functional connectivity between ventromedial prefrontal cortex and lower level regions (e.g. somatosensory cortex) in individuals with ASD during these self- representation tasks.

Previous studies identified the right inferior parietal lobe, along with frontopolar and somatosensory regions [36,37] as critical for distinguishing between self and other. Additional data [e.g. 38] demonstrate that SI and SII cortices, which contribute to the mirror-neuron system, are also crucial for preserving a sense of self.

3.3. Body awareness, sense of agency

Knowing oneself and knowing one's body are closely related concepts. In his review on body image and the self, Goldenberg [39] argues that the acquisition of body image is not innate but acquired through experiences of one's own and other bodies. Likewise, Jordan and Powell [40] believe that a body concept develops from interacting with others. Anecdotal reports indicate that some children and adults with autism have an insecure body image or totally lack body awareness. Russell [41] suggested that the 'body schemas of persons with autism are poorly specified' resulting in an atypical experience of agency. A sense of agency is a central aspect of human self-consciousness and refers to the experience of oneself as the agent of ones actions. Based on his executive function account of impaired action monitoring Russell [42] put forward the hypothesis that individuals with autism are impaired in distinguishing between self and others. In contrast, a recent study by Williams and Happè [43] suggests that individuals with ASD are aware of their agency as indicated by their ability to monitor their own actions.

Support for a dominant role of the right hemisphere in the above processes is substantial. The right posterior parietal lobe is generally associated with spatial and bodily awareness [44,45]. Activation of right inferior parietal lobe correlates with a sense of ownership in action execution [46]. Additional research evidence [47] based on transcranial magnetic stimulation (TMS) supports the significance of the right temporo-parietal junction in the maintenance of a coherent sense of one's body.

3.4. Theory of mind, emotions and self-awareness

An essential component of self-awareness is the ability to be aware of other minds. A multitude of studies have provided evidence that theory of mind is lacking or delayed in ASD, or develops differently than in neurotypicals [for a substantive review see 48]. Deficits in mindreading may also affect the ability to reflect on one's own mental states [49] resulting in diminished self-awareness. There is some evidence suggesting that the ability to think about one's own thoughts depends on the same cognitive and neural processes as mindreading [50]. Equally, emotions play an important role in self-awareness. The development of the capacity to experience, communicate and regulate emotions is considered to be the most important event in infancy [51]. One of the main characteristics of autism is lack of empathy and emotional engagement with others [52,53]. Children with autism have difficulties with interpreting emotions, are deficient in processing their own emotional experiences and pay little attention to emotional stimuli in general [e.g. 54-57]. Due to this inability to empathize and emotionally engage with others individuals with ASD are totally focussed on their own interests and concerns.

A network of structures important for theory of mind processing includes the superior temporal sulcus and the adjacent temporo-parietal junction, the temporal poles and the medial prefrontal cortex [58; see also 59 for a review). Research evidence implicated the RH in theory of mind reasoning across various tasks [60, 61]. The neural substrates for emotions and empathy are complex [62] involving amygdala, ventral medial prefrontal cortex. Recent imaging studies point to an involvement of a 'mirror neuron circuit' for empathy [63,64].

3.5. Egocentrism/Allocentrism

In apparent contrast to the mentalizing impairment even among very high functioning individuals with ASD is their often-documented increased sense of self or total focus on the self [65,66,67] that is also reflected in numerous biographical accounts. The term 'autism' is derived from the Greek word 'autos' ('self') and since Kanner's time this focus on the self as atypical applies to all individuals with ASD. Extreme egocentricity was one of the diagnostic criteria for Asperger Syndrome proposed by Gillberg & Gillberg [68]. Frith and de Vignemont [69] suggest that there are differences to reading other minds depending on whether the other person can be understood using an 'egocentric' or an 'allocentric' standpoint. From an egocentric point of view other people are understood only relative to the self whereas from an allocentric stance the mental state of a person is independent from the self. These theorists suggest that individuals with ASD suffer from an imbalance between both point of views, 'they are unable to connect an egocentric to an allocentric stance and can only adopt extreme forms of either' [70]. This very detailed analysis of mindreading further illustrates the different and unique aspects of awareness of self and others in individuals with ASD.

3.6. Self awareness across time

Awareness that we are the same person across time, also defined as temporally extended self-awareness [71] is an essential part of one's self-concept. Although the results of two recent studies [72,73] indicate that individuals with ASD have undiminished temporally extended self-awareness as assessed by the delayed self-recognition task, this task may not adequately measure self-awareness as suggested by Lind & Bowler [74]. Indirect evidence suggests that temporally extended self-awareness is impaired in ASD based on their problems with theory of mind as well as some aspects of temporal cognition [75]. Alternative explanations are the autobiographic memory difficulties [76] and also the well-documented language impairments in ASD. Language is a medium with which we monitor ourselves and it allows us to experience past, present and future [77].

3.7. Language and awareness of self

Conceptions about oneself and others develop from an early age and depend largely on the emergence of language. At around 18 months of age children start referring to themselves as 'I' and begin using the word 'you' for others, indicating a further development in their self-other awareness. According to Kircher and David [78] 'the symbolic presentation of the self in language is the personal pronoun I'. Language difficulties such as pronoun reversal, use of third person perspective, impoverished inner speech, and impaired narrative have a negative effect on mental processes and also restrict certain aspects of self-awareness.

There is substantial clinical and research evidence of impaired pragmatic language use in children with ASD as indicated by pronoun reversal errors ('I'/'me/'you') [79-82] reflecting general difficulties with their sense of self, as well as problems in self-other differentiation.

Peeters et al. [83] suggested that the reason children with autism sometimes communicate from a third-person perspective instead of a first- vis-à-vis second person perspective is that in contrast to typically developing children they possess a non-social basis of self-other categorization. Use of a third person perspective also has consequences for attribution of mental states, and mentalizing ability in general. As argued by Northoff and Heinzel [84] a third person perspective is an indication of a fragmented image of self and other. Adults with

ASD also appear to have difficulties with first person pronoun usage [85]. Of particular interest might be the fact, that Hans Asperger often used to refer to himself from a third person perspective [86].

A fundamental role in self-awareness is attributed to inner speech [87] that is impaired in ASD [88]. When asked about the nature of their thoughts, a group of adults with Asperger syndrome reported mainly images and actions as their only inner experience and made no reference to inner speech or emotions [89]. Many individuals with ASD are visual thinkers and rely heavily on visualization to process information [90].

A recent fMRI study [91] provided evidence of underintegration of language and imaging in autism by showing that individuals with ASD are more reliant on visualization to support language comprehension. These authors suggest that cortical underconnectivity is the reason for the lack of synchronization between linguistic and imaginal processing in autism. Supporting these findings are the results of an imaging study on daydreaming [92] indicating that autistic individuals do not 'daydream' about themselves or other people. This study also points to a link between daydreaming and the construction of self and self-awareness.

In summary, language is of fundamental significance to self-awareness and necessary for forming a clear identity of self and others. Another important dimension in the formation of the self that is also dependent on language is autobiographical memory as well as the construct of a narrative self.

3.8. Autobiographical memory

Many influential theorists [93,94] associate the development of self with the emergence of autobiographical or episodic memory. The components necessary for a fully functioning autobiographical memory are a basic memory system, spoken or signed language, understanding and production of narrative, temporal understanding, self-awareness and theory of mind [95]. Autobiographical memory not only depends on these cognitive constructs but is also specifically concerned with events that have specific meaning to the individual. This personal significance evolves through emotions and motivations that are constructed in interaction with others. Autobiographical disturbances can arise from combined deficits in the realms of memory, emotion and self-related processing which are intricately connected, both behaviourally and neurologically [96].

The majority of components that make up an autobiographic memory system are impaired in autism. There is significant evidence that individuals with ASD have circumscribed episodic memory impairments, e.g. they have an impaired recall for personally experienced events [97-101]. As suggested by Millward et al [102] individuals with ASD remember real-life episodes less well than other people because they have no 'experiencing self'. Wheeler et al [103] in their investigation of episodic memory in autism concluded that remembering of personal events requires the 'highest form of consciousness, autonoetic consciousness (self-knowing), which is dependent of self-awareness'.

The prevailing view is that episodic memory is created in the neocortex and subsequently stored in the medial-temporal lobes and after a time becomes independent and is distributed in neocortical networks [104]. Whereas the left temporal lobe is dominant for the acquisition of new verbal information, episodic information involves mainly the right fontal lobes [105, 106]. Neuroimaging studies provide evidence for right frontal involvement in the processing of autobiographic memories [e.g. 107]. The RH is especially important for memories with emotional contents.

3.9. The narrative self

Many theorists [e.g. 108, 109] have highlighted the importance of the narrative self and argued that the autobiographical self is a similar construct as the narrative self. Individuals create their own identity by constructing autobiographical narratives or life stories [110]. The benefits of a personal or narrative self are significant; a narrative mediates self-understanding and creates coherence out of life's experiences. Narrative emerges early in development and narrative and self are inseparable [111]. The creation of a narrative self depends on various cognitive capacities, including working memory, self-awareness, episodic memory and reflective metacognition, a sense of agency, the ability to attribute action to oneself together with a capacity for temporal integration of events, a fully functioning pronoun system, an ability to differentiate between self and non-self as well as a sense of one's own body that is based on proprioceptive-motor processes [112].

The mechanisms responsible for each of the above dimensions are impaired in autism and as a consequence individuals with ASD have great difficulties in constructing a self-narrative. If autobiographical material cannot be provided, the narrative is disoriented and confused and in many cases is no narrative at all but only confabulation [113], which is often the case in autism. As a result, the narrative of individuals with ASD, and the self that is represented in this narrative, is quite vague and not representing the true self. Research evidence confirms deficits in narrative abilities in individuals with ASD [114-116].

Language and symbolic functions are localized in the left hemisphere, whereas narrative abilities are considered to be a function of the right hemisphere. There is a significant evidence for RH contribution to social language and many of the functions associated with autobiographic memory specifically those with emotional contents. In addition, narrative organisation depends on coordination of activity among various brain regions [117] and as suggested by Belmonte [118] malfunction in neural connectivity may be the underlying problem with autistic narrative.

To summarize, there is substantial evidence that the main components of self-awareness including self recognition, self-other differentiation, body awareness, theory of mind, intersubjectivity, emotion processing, language (pronoun reversal, inner speech, third person perspective), autobiographical memory and narrative self are impaired in ASD. Our review of neural substrates underlying these processes has highlighted the significance of the Right Hemisphere.

4. Self neuropathology in ASD

From a neural point of view the self can be viewed as a complex and dynamic representation consisting of multiple brain networks [119, 120]. The origins of self begin in infancy and over the first several years of life normally developing children acquire an understanding of different dimensions of self and other. Deviant development in autism is likely to result in a cascade of developmental impairments including dysfunctional self-related processes as outlined above. Various brain regions have been indicated in the pathogenesis of autism including frontal lobes [e.g., 121] cerebellum [122], parietal lobes [123], hippocampus [124] and amygdala [125]. The extent of anatomical and functional abnormalities in autism points to a possible core dysfunction in neural processing. In addition, the vast amount of potential genetic risk factors suggests that multiple or all-emerging functional brain areas are affected during early development [126]. This theory is supported by widespread growth abnormalities in the brain of children with autism [127, 128].

In the following sections we will explore three neural theories implicated in the development of an atypical or different sense of self in individuals with ASD. Apart from the involvement of the RH in self-related processes a dysfunctional mirror neuron system as well as abnormal connectivity may have a role to play in the atypical developmental trajectories in ASD.

4.1. Right hemisphere hypothesis

The prefrontal cortex plays a vital role in the development of the self as it generates a sense of self and facilitates many links with other parts of the brain. Cognitive neuroscience studies have shown that the RH plays a special role in personal relatedness, which is intimately linked to the development of the self. Based largely on recent neuroimaging research evidence an increasing number of cognitive neuroscientists have emphasized the specific role of the RH in self-related functions [129-132]. Specifically the right dorsomedial prefrontal cortex seems to play a critical role in the development of models of the self [133]. This has been confirmed by several imaging studies, including a recent study of self-evaluation [134]. As described in the previous paragraphs there is substantial research evidence that the RH may be dominant for self-awareness and self-related functions. The psychiatrist and philosopher Iain McGilchrist [135] provided an extensive exploration of the dominance of the RH in self-related processes.

Elsewhere, Lyons and Fitzgerald [136] put forward the theory that RH impairment leads to a dysfunctional self-development in ASD. There is substantial research evidence linking Asperger syndrome to right hemisphere dysfunction [e.g. 137, 138]. The RH is dominant in the first years of human life when the major brain development during critical periods takes place. Results of a cerebral metabolism study in children (aged between 18 days to 12 years) showed that the RH is prominently activated, suggesting that the RH develops earlier than the LH [139]. The RH in implicated during early social interactions [140] including early attachment processes [141], maternal face and voice recognition [142] as well as the ability to view others in a similar way as the self [143]. The developing self depends on relations with others and these early experiences are vital for the maturation of the right brain system. Substantial behavioural evidence of infants who later developed autism is supporting the theory of disrupted intersubjective behaviour. We argue that impairments in neurobiology affecting particularly the RH both cause and interact with defects in personal relatedness and later developing self processes.

4.2. Abnormal connectivity

The 'Abnormal Neural Connectivity Theory' proposes that autism is a distributed system-wide brain disorder that restricts the coordination and integration among various brain areas. The original positron emission tomography (PET) study by Horwitz et al. [144] found reduced correlations among frontal cortex, parietal and other brain regions and suggested that autism involves impairment in functional connectivity between frontal cortex and other brain systems. More recent studies proposed that autism is a disorder of neural underconnectivity [145], overconnectivity [146, 147] or both under and overconnectivity in which local connectivity may be relatively dense whereas long-range connectivity between brain regions may be reduced or abnormally patterned [146-151].

Studies of the cerebral cortex in autism show abnormalities of synaptic and columnar structure. Cortical minicolumns are fundamental units of cerebral cortical information processing. Examination of neurons revealed abnormalities in the size of cortical minicolumns particularly in the frontal and temporal lobes in ASD [152, 153] that could alter overall levels of connectivity within the brain. These findings are in accordance with the observed white matter abnormalities reported particularly in people with ASD [154]. A recent study using functional connectivity MRI (fcMRI) [155] provided further evidence of atypical enhanced functional connectivity suggesting that abnormal connectivity may be linked to developmental brain growth disturbances in autism.

These studies suggest that connectivity among diverse brain areas may be the core problem in autism. In autism the network connectivity through which various brain areas communicate with each other are limited, particularly the connections to the frontal cortex [156] which is dominant for self-related processing particularly in the RH. The network model of the self proposed by Stuss et al. [157] suggests that the self is hierarchically organized, with the highest level of the self involved in self-awareness being subserved by frontal lobes. Early developmental impairments in minicolumnar microcircuitry in the frontal cortex in autism could be the reason for the deficits found in higher order frontal processes [158] which are likely to result in fragmented self awareness and identity formation in autism.

4.3. Mirror neuron system

Another recent neural theory of autism suggests that a dysfunctional mirror neuron system may be fundamental to the aetiology of autism [159, 160]. The existence of mirror neurons in humans has been demonstrated by a number of EEG and imaging studies [e.g. 161]. Mirror neurons are activated in relation both to specific actions performed by self and matching actions performed by others, providing a potential bridge between minds [162] and might have a role to play in self related processes. Mirror neurons may enable us to understand the actions of others by mapping the actions of other people to our own motor system and so allow a shared representation of actions. In addition to understanding the action of others this so-called 'mirroring' might also allow the automatic experience of the intention and emotion of the other person as suggested by Kaplan and Iacoboni [163].

Research has demonstrated that mirror neuron activity correlates with empathy [164] and social competence in general [165]. It has been suggested that mirror neurons are a prerequisite for the normal development of self-recognition, imitation, theory of mind, empathy, intersubjectivity and language [166, 167]. Furthermore, mirror neurons are likely to play a central role in self-awareness. To quote Ramachandran and Oberman [168] 'they may enable humans to see themselves as others see them, which may be an essential ability for self-awareness and introspection' (p.41). Developmental data suggest that there is higher imitative behaviour in children that can self-recognise, possibly facilitated by mirror neurons, in contrast to those who cannot [169]. Providing support for a RH hypothesis in self-related functions are recent imaging studies [170, 171] indicating that a frontoparietal 'mirror' network is associated with self-recognition processes.

Several recent functional brain-imaging studies have found evidence of mirror neuron dysfunction in individuals with ASD in social mirroring tasks [172], motor facilitation [173], and imitation [174]. A fMRI study [175] revealed that individuals with autism showed a different pattern of brain activity during cognitive tasks relating to self-referential processing. The authors concluded that a core deficit in autism might be related to the construction of a sense of self in its relation with others. Echoing Hobson [176] Iacoboni [177] suggests that primary intersubjectivity is the basis for the development of the neural systems associated with internal and external self-related processes. Failure or abnormal development of a fully functioning mirror neuron system in the autistic infant is likely to result in a cascade of developmental impairments including dysfunctional self-related processes.

5. Conclusion

The centrality of an impaired sense of self in autism has been the focus of research for many decades. The development of self-awareness is a complex process that involves integration of information from many sources and coordination across the brain systems involved in self-related concepts. A sense of self emerges from the activity of the brain in interaction with other selves. There is substantial evidence that early deficits in self-development including impaired relations with others result in a fragmented and atypical sense of self in ASD. In this review we have presented evidence that a great majority of self-related processes that are mediated to a significant extent by the right hemisphere are impaired in individuals with ASD. Additional lines of investigation indicate that an unintegrated sense of self in autism is also potentially associated with abnormal functional connectivity and an impaired mirror neuron system. Consequences of this atypical sense of self are the well-documented impairments individuals with ASD experience in the social and communication domain. In contrast, there have been suggestions that this different sense of self might be a contributory factor to the significant talents and special skills present in a majority of individuals with ASD. Happè & Vital [178] put forward the notion that diminished self-awareness in ASD might be advantageous in the development of these special gifts.

Author details

Viktoria Lyons[1] and Michael Fitzgerald[2]

*Address all correspondence to: viktorialyons@yahoo.co.uk

1 Blackrock, Co. Dublin, Ireland

2 Trinity College Dublin, Ireland

References

[1] Kircher T, David AS. Introduction: The Self And Neuroscience. In: Kircher T, David A.S. (eds) The Self in Neuroscience and Psychiatry, Cambridge: Cambridge University Press; 2003. p2.

[2] Kanner L. Autistic Disturbances of Affective Contact. Nervous Child 1943;2: 217-50.

[3] Asperger H. Frühkindlicher Autismus, Medizinische Klinik 1974;69: 2024-27.

[4] Cohen DJ. The pathology of the Self in primary childhood autism and Gilles de la Tourette Syndrome. Psychiatric Clinics of North America 1980; 3 (3): 383-402.

[5] Lutz J. Zum Verstaendnis Des Autismus Infantum Als Einer Ich-Bewusstseins-, Ich-Aktivitaets- Und Ich-Einpraegungsstoerung. Acta Paedopsychiatrica 1968; 35, 161.

[6] Powell S, Jordan R. Being Subjective About Autistic Thinking And Learning To Learn. Educational Psychology 1993;13: 359-370.

[7] Frith U. Autism: Explaining The Enigma. Oxford: Blackwell; 1989, 2nd Edition; 2003.

[8] Hobson RP. On The Origins Of Self And The Case Of Autism. Development And Psychopathology 1990;2: 163-81.

[9] Hobson RP, Meyer JA. Foundations For Self And Other: A Study In Autism. Developmental Science 2005;8: 481-91.

[10] Stern DN. The Interpersonal World Of The Infant. New York: Basic Books; 1985.

[11] Neisser U. Five kinds of self-knowledge. Philosophical Psychology 1988;1(1): 35-58.

[12] Dahlgren SO, Gillberg C. Symptoms in the first two years of life. A preliminary population study of infantile autism. European Archives of Psychiatric and Neurological Science 1989; 283: 169-74.

[13] Nadig AS, Ozonoff S, Young GS, Rozga A, Sigman M, Rogers SJ. A Prospective Study Of Response To Name In Infants At Risk For Autism. Archives Pediatric Adolescent Medicine 2007;161: 378-83.

[14] Osterling J, Dawson G. Early Recognition Of Children With Autism: A Study Of First Birthday Home Videotapes. Journal Of Autism And Developmental Disorders 1994;24: 247-53.

[15] Baron-Cohen S, Cos A, Bird G, Swettenham J, Nightingale N, Morgan K, Drew A. Charman T. Psychological markers in the detection of autism in infancy in a large population. British Journal of Psychiatry 1996;16: 158-63.

[16] Dawson G, Adams A. Imitation and social responsiveness in autistic children. Journal of Abnormal Child Psychology 1984;12 (2): 209-26.

[17] Mundy P, Crowson M. Joint Attention And Early Communication: Implications For Intervention With Autism. Journal Of Autism And Developmental Disorders 1997;6: 653-76.

[18] Hobson RP. Autism And The Development Of Mind. Hillsdale, NJ: Lawrence Erlbaum; 1993.

[19] Hobson, 1990.

[20] Gallup GG. Jr. Chimpanzees: Self-Recognition. Science 1970;167: 86-87.

[21] Lewis M., Ramsay D. Intentions, Consciousness And Pretend Play. In: Zelazo PD, Astington JW, Olson DR (eds) Developing Theories Of Intention: Social Understanding And Self-Control. Mahwah, NJ: Erlbaum; 1999. p77-94,

[22] Dawson G, McKissick FC. Self-recognition in autistic children. Journal of Autism and Developmental Disorders 1984;17: 383-94.

[23] Keenan JP, Christiana W, Malcolm S, Johnson A. Mirror-Self Recognition In Autism And Asperger's Syndrome: Implications For Neurological Correlates'. Poster Presented At The Eleventh Annual Cognitive Neuroscience Society Meeting, San Francisco. CA., April 2004.

[24] Pierce K., Muller R-A., Ambrose J., Allen G., Courchesne E. Face Processing Occurs Outside The Fusiform 'Face Area' In Autism: Evidence From Functional MRI'. Brain 2001;124: 2059-73.

[25] Keenan JP, McCutcheon NB, Pascual-Leone A. Functional Magnetic Resonance Imaging And Event Related Potential Suggest Right Prefrontal Activation For Self-Related Processing. Brain And Cognition 2001;47: 87-91.

[26] Critchley HD, Daly EM, Bullmore ET. Et Al. The functional neuroanatomy of social behavior. Changes in cerebral blood flow when people with autistic disorder process facial expressions. Brain 2000;123: 2203-12.

[27] Pierce et al., (2001).

[28] Hobson (1990).

[29] Hobson & Meyer (2005).

[30] Murray D, Lesser M. Lawson W. Attention, Monotropism And The Diagnostic Criteria For Autism. Autism. The International Journal Of Research And Practice 2005;9 (2): 139-56.

[31] Williams D. Autism And Sensing. The Unlost Instinct. London: Jessica Kingsley; 1998.

[32] Chiu PH, Kayali MA, Kishida KT, Tomlin D, Klinger LG, Klinger MR, Montague PR. Self Responses along cingulate cortex reveal quantitative neural phenotype for high-functioning autism. Neuron 2008;57: 463-73.

[33] Tomlin D, Kayali M A, King-Casas B, Anen D, Camerer CF, Et Al. Agent-Specific Responses In The Cingulated Cortex During Economic Exchanges. Science 2006;5776: 1047-50.

[34] Chiu et al. (2008).

[35] Lombardo MV, Chakrabarti B, Bullmore ET, Sadek SA, Pasco G, Wheelwright SJ, Suckling J, MRC AIMS Consortium, Baron-Cohen S. (2009). Atypical Neural Self-Representation in Autism. Brain 2009. http://brain.oxfordjournals.org/cgi/content/abstract/awp306v1(accessed 19 January 2010)

[36] Ruby P, Decety J. How Would You Feel Versus How Do You Think She Would Feel? A Neuroimaging Study On Perspective-Taking With Social Emotions. Journal Of Cognitive Neuroscience 2003;16: 988-99.

[37] Decety J, Sommerville JA. Shared representations between self and other: A social cognitive neuroscience view. Trends in Cognitive Science 2003;7: 527-33.

[38] Avikainen S, Forss N, Hair R. Modulated activation of the human SI and SII cortices during observation of hand actions. Neuron 2002;15: 640-6.

[39] Goldenberg G. Body Image And The Self. In: Feinberg TE, Keenan JP (eds.) The Lost Self. Pathologies Of The Brain And Identity. Oxford: Oxford University Press; 2005. p81-99.

[40] Jordan R, Powell S. Understanding And Teaching Children With Autism. Chichester: Wiley; 1995.

[41] Russell J. How Executive Disorders Can Bring About An Inadequate 'Theory Of Mind'. In: Russell J (Ed.) Autism As An Executive Disorder. Oxford: Oxford University Press. 1997.p281.

[42] Russell (1997).

[43] Williams D, Happé F. Pre-Conceptual Aspects Of Self-Awareness In Autism Spectrum Disorder: The Case Of Action Monitoring. Journal Of Autism And Developmental Disorders 2009;39: 251-9.

[44] Mesulam MM. Principles Of Behavioral And Cognitive Neurology (2nd Ed.), Oxford: Oxford University Press; 2000.

[45] Devinsky O. Right Cerebral Hemisphere Dominance for a Sense of Corporeal and Emotional Self. Epilepsy & Behaviour 2000;1: 60-73.

[46] Farrer C, Franck N, Georgieff N, Frith CD, Decety J, Et Al. Modulating The Experience Of Agency: A Positron Emission Tomography Study. Neuroimage 2003;18: 324-33.

[47] Tsakiris M, Constantine M, Haggard P. The Role Of Right Temporo-Parietal Junction In Maintaining A Coherent Sense Of One's Body. Neuropsychologia 2008;46: 3014-18.

[48] Saxe R, Baron-Cohen, S. Editorial: The Neuroscience Of Theory Of Mind. In: R. Saxe R, Baron-Cohen S. (eds.) Theory Of Mind. A Special Issue Of The Journal Social Neuroscience. Hove: Psychology Press; 2007.

[49] Frith U, Happè F. Theory Of Mind And Self Consciousness: What It Is Like To Be Autistic? Mind & Language 1999;14: 1-22.

[50] Happè F. Theory Of Mind And The Self. In: Ledoux J, Debiec J, Moss H. (eds) The Self: From Soul To Brain, Annals Of The New York Academy Of Sciences 2003;1001: 134-144.

[51] Schore AN. Affect Dysregulation And Disorders of The Self. New York: Ww. Norton & Company; 2003.

[52] Baron-Cohen S. Wheelwright S. The Empathy quotient: An investigation of adults with Asperger syndrome or high functioning autism, and normal sex differences. Journal of Autism and Developmental Disorders 2004;34: 163-75.

[53] Hobson (1993).

[54] Hobson RP. The Autistic Child's Appraisal Of Expressions Of Emotion. Journal Of Child Psychology And Psychiatry 1986; 27: 321-42.

[55] Yirmiya N., Sigman M., Kasari C., Mundy P. Empathy And Cognition In High Functioning Children With Autism. Child Development 1992;63: 150-60.

[56] Baron-Cohen S., Wheelwright S., Joliffe T. Is there a 'language of the eyes'? Evidence from normal adults and adults with autism or Asperger syndrome. Visual Cognition 1997;4: 311-31.

[57] Gaigg SB, Bowler DM. Free Recall And Forgetting Of Emotionally Arousing Words In Autism Spectrum Disorder. Neuropsychologia 2008;46: 2336-43.

[58] Frith CD, Frith U. The Neural Basis Of Mentalizing. Neuron 2006;50: 531-34.

[59] Saxe & Baron-Cohen (2007).

[60] Happé F., Brownell H., Winner E. Acquired Theory Of Mind Impairments Following Right Hemisphere Stroke. Cognition 1999;70: 211-40.

[61] Shamay-Tsoory SG, Tomer R, Berger BD., Goldsher D,Aharon-Peretz, J. Impaired "Affective Theory Of Mind" Is Associated With Right Ventromedial Prefrontal Damage. Cognitive And Behavioural Neurology 2005;18: 55-67.

[62] Chakrabarti B, Bullmore E, Baron-Cohen S. (2007) 'Empathizing with basic emotions: Common and discrete neural substrates. In: Saxe R, Baron-Cohen S. (eds) Theory of Mind. A special issue of the Journal Social Neuroscience. Hove: Psychology Press; 2007. p. 364-384.

[63] Keysers C., Perrett I. Demystifying Social Cognition: A Hebbian Perspective. Trends In Cognitive Science 2004;8: 501-7.

[64] Rizzolatti G, Craighero L. The Mirror-Neuron Sys tem. Annual Reviews Of Neuroscience 2004; 27: 169-92.

[65] Kanner (1943).

[66] Asperger H. Die 'autistischen Psychopathen' im Kindesalter. Archiv für Psychiatrie and Nervenkrankheiten 1944;117: 78-136.

[67] Baron-Cohen, S. (2005) 'Autism – 'Autos': Literally, a Total Focus on the Self?' In: Feinberg TE., Keenan JP (eds.) The Lost Self. Pathologies of the Brain and Identity. Oxford: Oxford University Press. p166-80.

[68] Gillberg IC, Gillberg C. Asperger Syndrome – Some Epidemiological Considerations: A Research Note. Journal Of Child Psychology And Psychiatry 1989;30: 631-38.

[69] Frith U, De Vignemont, F. Egocentrism, Allocentrism, And Asperger Syndrome. Consciousness And Cognition 2005;14: 719-38.

[70] Frith U, De Vignemont F. (2005)

[71] Moore C, Lemmon K. The Self In Time: Developmental Perspectives. Hillsdale, NJ, Usa: Erlbaum; 2001.

[72] Nielsen M., Suddendorf T., Dissanayake C. Imitation And Self-Recognition In Autism. In: Rogers S., Williams JW. (Eds) Imitation And The Development Of The Social Mind: Autism And Typical Development. New York: Guilford Press; 2006. p138-56.

[73] Lind SE, Bowler DM. Delayed Self-Recognition In Children With Autism Spectrum Disorder. Journal Of Autism And Developmental Disorders 2009;39 (4): 643-650.

[74] Lind SE, Bowler DM. (2009).

[75] Boucher J, Pons F, Lind S, Williams D. Temporal cognition in children with autistic spectrum disorders: Tests of diachronic thinking. Journal of Autism and Developmental Disorders 2007;37: 1413-29.

[76] Lind SE, Bowler DM. Episodic Memory And Autonoetic Consciousness In Autistic Spectrum Disorders: The Roles Of Self-Awareness, Representational Abilities And Temporal Cognition. In: Boucher J, Bowler DM. (eds), Memory In Autism: Theory And Evidence. Cambridge: Cambridge University Press; 2008. p166-188.

[77] Beitman BD, Nair J, Viamontes GI. 'Why Self-Awareness?' In: Beitman BD, J. Nair J. (eds.) Self-Awareness Deficits in Psychiatric Patients. Neurobiology, Assessment, and Treatment. New York: W.W. Norton & Company; 2004. p3-23.

[78] Kircher T, David AS. (2003) p3.

[79] Kanner L. (1943).

[80] Tager-Flusberg, H. Current Theory And Research On Language And Communication In Autism. Journal Of Autism And Developmental Disorders 1996;26: 169-172.

[81] Hobson (1990).

[82] Jordan R, Powell S. (1995).

[83] Peeters G, Grobben G, Hendrickx,A., Van Den Eede S, Verlinden K. Self-Other And Third-Person Categorization In Normal And Autistic Children. Developmental Science 2003. 6: 166-172.

[84] Northoff G, Heinzel A. The Self In Philosophy, Neuroscience And Psychiatry: An Epistemic Approach', In: T. Kircher T., David A. (eds.) The Self In Neuroscience And Psychiatry. Cambridge: Cambridge University Press; 2003. p40-55.

[85] Lombardo MV, Barnes JL, Wheelwright SJ, Baron-Cohen S. Self-Referential Cognition And Empathy In Autism. PloS One 2007,2: e883.

[86] Lyons V, Fitzgerald M. Asperger Syndrome – A Gift Or A Curse? New York: Nova Science Publishers; 2007.

[87] Siegrist M. Inner Speech As A Cognitive Process Mediating Self-Consciousness And Inhibiting Self-Deception. Psychology Report 1995;76: 259-265.

[88] Whitehouse A.JO, Maybery MT, Durkin K. Inner Speech Impairments In Autism. Journal Of Child Psychology And Psychiatry 2006;47: 857-65.

[89] Hurlburt R, Happé F, Frith U. Sampling The Form Of Inner Experience In Three Adults With Asperger's Syndrome. Psychological Medicine 1994;24: 385-95.

[90] Grandin T. Thinking In Pictures: And Other Reports From My Life With Autism. New York: Vintage Books; 1995.

[91] Kana RK, Keller TA, Cherkassky VL, Minshew NJ, Just MA. Sentence Comprehension In Autism: Thinking In Pictures With Decreased Functional Connectivity. Brain 2006;129: 2484-93.

[92] Kennedy DP, Redcay E, Courchesne E. Failing To Deactivate: Resting Functional Abnormalities In Autism. Proceedings Of The National Academy Of Science USA 2006;103: 8275-80.

[93] Perner J. Episodic Memory: Essential Distinctions And Developmental Implications. In: Moore C, Lemmon K.(Eds.) The Self In Time: Developmental Perspectives. Hillsdale NJ: Erlbaum; 2001. p181-202.

[94] Wheeler MA. Episodic Memory And Autonoetic Awareness. In: Tulving E, Craik FIM. (eds.) Oxford Handbook Of Memory. New York: Oxford University Press; 2000. p597-625.

[95] Nelson K, Fivush R. The Emergence Of Autobiographical Memory: A Social Cultural Developmental Theory. Psychological Review 2004;111: 486-511.

[96] Fujiwara E, Markowitsch HJ. Autobiographical Disorders. In: Feinberg TE, Keenan JP. (eds.) The Lost Self. Pathologies Of The Brain And Identity, Oxford: Oxford University Press; 2005. p65-80.

[97] Bowler DM, Gardiner JM, Grice SJ. Episodic memory and remembering in adults with Asperger syndrome. Journal of Autism and Developmental Disorders 2000;30: 295-304, p. 295.

[98] Millward C, Powell S, Messer D, Jordan R. Recall For Self And Other In Autism: Children's Memory For Events Experienced By Themselves And Their Peers. Journal For Autism And Developmental Disorders 2000;30: 15-28.

[99] Gardiner, J. M. Bowler, D. M, Grice SJ. Further Evidence Of Preserved Priming And Impaired Recall In Adults With Asperger's Syndrome. Journal Of Autism And Developmental Disorder 2003;33 (3) 250-69.

[100] Crane L, Goddard L. Episodic and semantic autobiographical memory in adults with Autism Spectrum Disorders. Journal of Autism and Developmental Disorders 2008; 38: 498-506.

[101] Boucher J, Bowler DM (eds) Memory in autism: theory and evidence. Cambridge: Cambridge University Press; 2008.

[102] Millward et al. (2000).

[103] Wheeler MA, Stuss DT, Tulving, E Toward A Theory Of Episodic Memory: The Frontal Lobes And Autonoetic Consciousness. Psychological Bulletin 1997;121: 331-54.

[104] Fink GR. In Search Of One's Own Past: The Neural Bases Of Autobiographical Memories. Brain 2003;126: 1509-10.

[105] Shallice T, Fletcher P, Frith C, Grasby P, Frackowiak R, Dolan R. Brain Regions Associated With Acquisition And Retrieval Of Verbal Episodic Memory. Nature 1994;368: 633-35.

[106] Tulving E, Kapur S, Craik F, Moskovitch M, Houle S. Hemispheric Encoding/Retrieval Asymmetry In Episodic Memory: Positron Emission Tomography Findings. Proceedings Of The National Academy Of Science USA 1994;91: 2016-20.

[107] Fink GR, Markowitsch HJ, Reinkemeier M, Bruckbauer T, Kessler J, Heiss W-D. Cerebral Representation Of One's Own Past: Neural Networks Involved In Autobiographical Memory', Journal of Neuroscience 1996;16: 4275-82.

[108] Bruner J. Kalmar DA. Narrative and metanarrative in the construction of self. In: Ferrari M, Sternberg RJ. (eds.) Self-Awareness: Its Nature and Development. New York: Guilford Press; 1988.

[109] Dennett D. Consciousness Explained. Boston: Little, Brown; 1991.

[110] Schechtman M. The Constitution Of Selves. Ithaca: Cornell University Press; 1996.

[111] Ochs E, Capps L. Narrating The Self. Annual Review Of Anthropology 1996;25: 19-43.

[112] Gallagher S. Self-Narrative In Schizophrenia. In: Kircher T, David A. (eds.) The Self In Neuroscience And Psychiatry. Cambridge: Cambridge University Press; 2003. p336-360.

[113] Gallagher (2003).

[114] Loveland K. Mcevoy R, Tunali B, Kelley ML. Narrative Story Telling In Autism And Down's Syndrome. British Journal of Developmental Psychology 1990;8: 9-23.

[115] Losh M, Capps L. Narrative Ability In Highfunctioning Children With Autism Or Asperger's Syndrome. Journal of Autism and Developmental Disorders 2003;33: 239-51.

[116] Colle L, Baron-Cohen S, Wheelwright S, Van Der Lely HK. Narrative discourse in adults with high-functioning Autism or Asperger Syndrome. Journal of Autism and Developmental Disorders 2008;38: 28-40.

[117] Tononi G, Sporns O, Edelman GM. Reentry And The Problem Of Integrating Multiple Cortical Areas: Simulation Of Dynamic Integration In The Visual System. Cerebral Cortex 1992; 2: 310-35.

[118] Belmonte M. Human, but more so: What the autistic brain tells us about the process of narrative. In: Osteen M. (ed.) Autism and representation. London: Routledge; 2008. p166-79.

[119] Viamontes GI, Beitman BD, Viamontes CT, Viamontes JA. Neural Circuits For Self-Awareness. Evolutionary Origins And Implementation In The Human Brain. In: Beit-

man BD, Nair J. (eds) Self-Awareness Deficits In Psychiatric Patients. Neurobiology, Assessment, And Treatment. New York: W.W. Norton & Company; 2004. p24-111.

[120] Decety & Somerville (2003).

[121] Aylward EH, Minshew NJ, Field, K, Sparks BF, Singh N. Effects of age on brain volume and head circumference in autism. Neurology 2002;59: 175-83.

[122] Courchesne E, Townsend J, Akshoomoff NA,Et al. A new finding: impairment in shifting attention in autistic and cerebellar patients. In: Broman SH, Grafman J. (eds) Atypical cognitive deficits in developmental disorders: implications for brain function. Hillsdale, N.J.: Lawrence Erlbaum Associates; 1994. p101-137.

[123] Courchesne E, Press G, Yeung-Courchesne, R. Parietal lobe abnormalities detected with MR in patients with infantile autism. American Journal of Roentgeneology 1993;160: 387-393.

[124] Saitoh O, Karnds,CM, Courchesne E. Development Of Hippocampal Formation From 2 To 42 Years: MRI Evidence Of Smaller Area Dentate In Autism. Brain 2001;124: 1317-24.

[125] Aylward EH, Minshew NJ, Goldstein G, Honeycutt NA., Augustine AM, Yates KO, Barta PE, Pearlson GD. MRI volumes of amygdala and hippocampus in non-mentally retarded autistic adolescents and adults. Neurology 1999;53: 2145-50.

[126] Müller RA. The Study Of Autism As A Distributed Disorder. Mental Retardation And Developmental Disabilities Research Review 2007;13(1): 85-95.

[127] Courchesne E, Karns CM, Davis HR, Ziccardi R, Carper RA. et al. Unusual brain growth patterns in early life in patients with autistic disorder: an MRI study. Neurology 2001;57: 245-54.

[128] Carper RA, Courchesne E. Localized enlargement of the frontal lobe in early autism. Biological Psychiatry 2005;57 (2): 126-33.

[129] Fossati P, Hevenor S, Graham SJ. Et Al. In Search Of The Emotional Self: An fMRI Study Using Positive And Negative Emotional Words. American Journal Of Psychiatry 2003;160: 1938-45.

[130] Keenan JP, Gallup GG, Jr., Falk D. The Face In The Mirror: The Search For The Origins Of Consciousness. New York: Harper Collins; 2003.

[131] Kircher & David (2001).

[132] Decety & Somervie (2003).

[133] Mega MS, Cummings JL. Frontal Subcortical Circuits: Anatomy And Function. In: Salloway SP, Malloy PF, Duffy JD. (Eds) The Frontal Lobes and Neuropsychiatric Illness. Washington, DC: American Psychiatric Publishing; 2001. p15-32.

[134] Fossati et al. (2003).

[135] McGilchrist I. The Master And His Emissary. The Divided Brain And The Making Of The Western World. New Haven and London: Yale University Press; 2010.

[136] Lyons V, Fitzgerald, M. 'Did Hans Asperger (1906-1980) Have Asperger Syndrome? Journal Of Autism And Developmental Disorder 2007;37: 2020-21.

[137] Klin A, Volkmar F, Sparrow, S, Cicchetti DV, Rourke BP. Validity and Neuropsychological Characterization of Asperger Syndrome: Convergence with Nonverbal Learning Disabilities Syndrome. Journal of Child Psychology and Psychiatry 1995; 36, 1127-1140.

[138] Gunter HL, Ghaziuddin M, Ellis HE. Asperger Syndrome: Test Of Right Hemisphere Functioning And Interhemispheric Communication. Journal Of Autism And Developmental Disorders 2002;32: 263-81.

[139] Chiron C, Jambaque I, Nabbout R, Lounes R, Syrota A., Dulac O. The right brain hemisphere is dominant in human infants. Brain 1997;120: 1057-1065.

[140] Geschwind N, Galaburda AM. Cerebral Lateralization: Biological Mechanisms, Associations, And Pathology. Boston: MIT Press; 1987.

[141] Schore AN. The Experience-Dependent Maturation Of A Regulatory System In The Orbital Prefrontal Cortex And The Origin Of Developmental Psychopathology'. Development and Psychopathology 1996;8: 59-87.

[142] Fernald A. Intonation And Communicative Interest In Mother's Speech To Infants: Is The Melody The Message? Child Development 1989;60: 1497-1510.

[143] Meltzoff AN, Brooks R. 'Like Me' As A Building Block For Understanding Other Minds: Bodily Acts, Attention And Intention. In Malle BF, Et Al (Eds) Intentions And Intentionality: Foundations For Social Cognition. Boston: MIT Press; 2001. p171-192.

[144] Horwitz, B, Rumsey JM, Grady C.L, Rapoport SI. The Cerebral Metabolic Landscape In Autism. Intercorrelations Of Regional Glucose Utilization. Archives Of Neurology 1988; 45: 749-755.

[145] Just MA, Cherkassky VL, Keller TA, Minshew N. Cortical Activation And Synchronization During Sentence Comprehension In High-Functioning Autism: Evidence Of Underconnectivity. Brain 2004;127 (8): 1811-21.

[146] Casanova MF. White matter volume increase and minicolumns in autism. Annals of Neurology 2004;56: 453-54.

[147] Mizuno A, Villalobos ME, Davies MM, Dahl BC, Müller RA. Partially Enhanced Talamocortical Functional Connectivity In Autism. Brain Research 2006;1104 (1): 160-174.

[148] Courchesne E, Pierce K. Why the frontal cortex in autism might be talking only to itself: local overconnectivity but long-distance disconnection. Current Opinion in Neurobiology 2005;15: 225-30.

[149] Belmonte M, Cook JEH, Anderson G, Rubinstein J, Greenough W, et al. Autism as a disorder of neural information processing: direction for research and targets for therapy. Molecular Psychiatry 2004a;9: 646-63.

[150] Kana et al. (2006).

[151] Just et al. (2007).

[152] Casanova MF, Buxhoeveden DP, Switala AE, Roy E. Minicolumnar pathology in autism. Neurology 2002a;58: 428-32.

[153] Casanova MF, Buxhoeveden DP, Switala AE, Roy E. Asperger's syndrome and cortical neuropathology. Journal of Child Neurology 2002b;17: 142-45.

[154] Keller TA., Kana RK, Just MA. A Developmental Study Of The Structural Integrity Of White Matter In Autism. Neuroreport 2007;18: 23-27.

[155] Turner KC, Frost L, Linsenbardt D, Mcilroy JR, Müller RA. Atypically Diffuse Functional Connectivity Between Caudate Nuclei And Cerebral Cortex. Behavioural And Brain Functions 2006;2: 34.

[156] Just MA., Cherkassky VL, Keller TA., Kana RK, Minshew N. Functional And Anatomical Cortical Underconnectivity In Autism: Evidence From A FMRI Study Of An Executive Function Task And Corpus Callosum Morphometry. Cerebral Cortex 2007;17: 951-61.

[157] Stuss DT, Picton TW, Alexander MP. Consciousness, Self-Awareness And The Frontal Lobes. In: Salloway SP, Malloy PF (eds.) The Frontal Lobes And Neuropsychiatric Illness. Washington, DC: American Psychiatric Publishing; 2001. P101-109.

[158] Courchesne & Pierce (2005).

[159] Williams JHG, Whiten A., Suddendorf T, Perrett DI. Imitation, Mirror Neurons And Autism. Neuroscience & Biobehavioral Reviews 2001;25: 287-95.

[160] Oberman LM, Ramachandran VS. The Simulating Social Mind: The Role Of The Mirror Neuron System And Simulation In The Social And Communicative Deficits In Autism Spectrum Disorders. Psychological Bulletin 2007;133(2): 310-27.

[161] Rizolatti & Craighero (2004).

[162] Williams et al. (2001).

[163] Kaplan JT, Iacoboni M. Getting A Grip On Other Minds: Mirror Neurons, Intention Understanding, And Cognitive Empathy. In: Saxe R, Baron-Cohen S. (eds.) Theory Of Mind. A Special Issue Of The Journal 'Social Neuroscience. Hove: Psychology Press; 2007. P175-183.

[164] Pfeifer J, Iacoboni M, Mazziotta JC, Dapretto M. Mirror neuron system activity correlates with empathy and interpersonal competence in children. Social Neuroscience 2006; 6 (3-4): 175-83.

[165] Kaplan & Iacoboni (2007).

[166] Oberman & Ramachandran (2007).

[167] Gallese V. The Roots Of Empathy: The Shared Hypothesis And The Neural Basis Of Intersubjectivity. Psychopathology 2003;36: 171-80.

[168] Ramachandran VS, Oberman LM. Broken Mirrors: A Theory Of Autism. Scientific American 2006; November, 39-45.

[169] Asendorpf JB, Baudonniere PM. Self-awareness and Other-awareness: Mirror self-recognition and synchronic imitation among unfamiliar peers. Developmental Psychology 1993;29: 88-95.

[170] Uddin LQ, Kaplan JT, Molnar-Szakacs I, Zaidel E, Iacoboni M. Self-Face Recognition Activates A Frontoparietal 'Mirror' Network In The Right Hemisphere: An Event-Related fMRI Study. Neuroimage 2005; 25: 926-35.

[171] Uddin LQ, Molnar-Szakacs I, Zaidel E, Iacoboni M. Rtms To The Right Inferior Parietal Area Disrupts Self-Other Discrimination. Social Cognitive And Affective Neuroscience 2006; 1, 65-71.

[172] Dapretto M, Davies MS, Pfeifer JH, Scott AA, Sigman,M. Bookheimer SY, Iacoboni M. Understanding emotions in others: mirror neuron dysfunction in children with autism spectrum disorders. Nature Neuroscience 2006;9(1): 28-30.

[173] Theoret H, Halligan E, Kobyashi M, Fregni F, Tager-Flusberg H, Pascual-Leone A. Impaired Motor Facilitation During Action Observation In Individuals With Autism Spectrum Disorder. Current Biology 2005;15: 84-85.

[174] Nishitani NA, Vikainen S, Hari R. Abnormal Imitation-Related Cortical Activation Sequences In Asperger's Syndrome. Annals Of Neurology 2004;55: 558-62.

[175] Kennedy et al. (2006).

[176] Hobson RP. The Intersubjective Foundations Of Thought. In Braten S. (ed.) Intersubjective Communication And Emotion In Early Ontogeny. Cambridge: Cambridge University Press; 1998. p283-296.

[177] Iacoboni, M. 'Failure To Deactivate In Autism: The Constitution Of Self And Other'. Retrieved October 7, 2006, From http://www.awares.org/conferences/

[178] Happè F, Vital P. 'What Aspects Of Autism Predispose To Talent?', In: Happè F, Frith U.(eds.) Autism And Talent. London: Philosophical Transactions of The Royal Society; 2009. p1369-1376.

Permissions

The contributors of this book come from diverse backgrounds, making this book a truly international effort. This book will bring forth new frontiers with its revolutionizing research information and detailed analysis of the nascent developments around the world.

We would like to thank Professor Michael Fitzgerald, for lending his expertise to make the book truly unique. He has played a crucial role in the development of this book. Without his invaluable contribution this book wouldn't have been possible. He has made vital efforts to compile up to date information on the varied aspects of this subject to make this book a valuable addition to the collection of many professionals and students.

This book was conceptualized with the vision of imparting up-to-date information and advanced data in this field. To ensure the same, a matchless editorial board was set up. Every individual on the board went through rigorous rounds of assessment to prove their worth. After which they invested a large part of their time researching and compiling the most relevant data for our readers. Conferences and sessions were held from time to time between the editorial board and the contributing authors to present the data in the most comprehensible form. The editorial team has worked tirelessly to provide valuable and valid information to help people across the globe.

Every chapter published in this book has been scrutinized by our experts. Their significance has been extensively debated. The topics covered herein carry significant findings which will fuel the growth of the discipline. They may even be implemented as practical applications or may be referred to as a beginning point for another development. Chapters in this book were first published by InTech; hereby published with permission under the Creative Commons Attribution License or equivalent.

The editorial board has been involved in producing this book since its inception. They have spent rigorous hours researching and exploring the diverse topics which have resulted in the successful publishing of this book. They have passed on their knowledge of decades through this book. To expedite this challenging task, the publisher supported the team at every step. A small team of assistant editors was also appointed to further simplify the editing procedure and attain best results for the readers.

Our editorial team has been hand-picked from every corner of the world. Their multi-ethnicity adds dynamic inputs to the discussions which result in innovative outcomes. These outcomes are then further discussed with the researchers and contributors who give their valuable feedback and opinion regarding the same. The feedback is then collaborated with the researches and they are edited in a comprehensive manner to aid the understanding of the subject.

Apart from the editorial board, the designing team has also invested a significant amount of their time in understanding the subject and creating the most relevant covers. They scrutinized every image to scout for the most suitable representation of the subject and create an appropriate cover for the book.

The publishing team has been involved in this book since its early stages. They were actively engaged in every process, be it collecting the data, connecting with the contributors or procuring relevant information. The team has been an ardent support to the editorial, designing and production team. Their endless efforts to recruit the best for this project, has resulted in the accomplishment of this book. They are a veteran in the field of academics and their pool of knowledge is as vast as their experience in printing. Their expertise and guidance has proved useful at every step. Their uncompromising quality standards have made this book an exceptional effort. Their encouragement from time to time has been an inspiration for everyone.

The publisher and the editorial board hope that this book will prove to be a valuable piece of knowledge for researchers, students, practitioners and scholars across the globe.

List of Contributors

Geneviève Nadon and Debbie Feldman
Université de Montréal and Center for Interdisciplinary Rehabilitation Research, Montreal, Quebec, Canada

Erika Gisel
Université de Montréal and Center for Interdisciplinary Rehabilitation Research, Montreal, Quebec, Canada
Faculty of Medicine, School of Physical & Occupational Therapy, McGill University, Canada

Olive Healy and Sinéad Lydon
National University of Ireland, Galway

Rudimar Riesgo and Michele Becker
Translational Research Group in Autism, (UFRGS) Federal University of Rio Grande do Sul, Porto Alegre, RS, Brazil
Child Neurology Unit, HCPA (Clinical Hospital of Porto Alegre), UFRGS, Porto Alegre, RS, Brazil

Carmem Gottfried
Translational Research Group in Autism, (UFRGS) Federal University of Rio Grande do Sul, Porto Alegre, RS, Brazil
Neuroglial Plasticity Laboratory, Department of Biochemistry, Postgraduate Program of Biochemistry, Institute of Basic Health Sciences, UFRGS, Porto Alegre, RS, Brazil

Fernanda Dreux Miranda Fernandes, Cibelle Albuquerque de La Higuera Amato, Danielle Azarias Defense-Netvral, Juliana Izidro Balestro and Daniela Regina Molini-Avejonas
Department of Phisical Therapy, Speech-Language Pathology and Audiology and Ocupational Therapy, School of Medicine, Universidade de São Paulo, São Paulo, Brazil

Liliana Maria Passerino
Graduate Program in Education (PPGEDU) and Computer Science and Education (PGIE) and the Interdisciplinary Center of Technologies in Education - CINTED/UFRGS, Computer Science and Education, Brazil

Maria Rosangela Bez
Interdisciplinary Center of Technologies in Education - CINTED/UFRGS, Brazil

Rubina Lal and Rakhee Chhabria
Department of Special Education, SNDT Women's University, Mumbai, India

Gunilla Thunberg
DART - Centre for AAC and Assistive Technology, Sahlgrenska University Hospital, Sweden

Viktoria Lyons and Michael Fitzgerald
Trinity College Dublin, Ireland